OSCEs in Psychiatry

Edited by Ranga Rao

Gaskell

© The Royal College of Psychiatrists 2005

Gaskell is an imprint of the Royal College of Psychiatrists, 17 Belgrave Square, London SW1X 8PG
http://www.rcpsych.ac.uk

British Library Cataloguing-in-Publication Data.
A catalogue record for this book is available from the British Library.
ISBN 1-904671-17-9

Distributed in North America by Balogh International Inc.

The views presented in this book do not necessarily reflect those of the Royal College
of Psychiatrists, and the publishers are not responsible for any error of omission or fact.

The Royal College of Psychiatrists is a registered charity (no. 228636).
Printed by Bell & Bain Limited, Thornliebank, Glasgow.

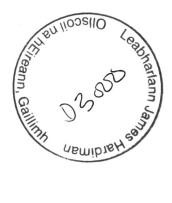

To my wife Natasha and children, Alekhia and Ujwal, for giving me the space and time.

Ranga Rao

Contents

Contributors

Anish Bahra, Consultant Neurologist, National Hospital for Neurology and Neurosurgery, Queen Square, London WC1N 3BG

Peter Bowie, Senior Lecturer in Old Age Psychiatry, Academic Unit of Psychiatry and Behavioural Sciences, University of Leeds, 15 Hyde Terrace, Leeds LS2 9LT

Nick Dunn, Consultant Psychiatrist, South London and Maudsley NHS Trust, Northover Mental Health Advice Centre, 102–104 Northover, Downham, Bromley BR1 5JX

Linda Gask, Reader in Community Psychiatry, University of Manchester, School of Primary Care, Rusholme Health Centre, Walmer Street, Manchester M14 5NP

Amanda Hukin, Specialist Registrar, General Adult Psychiatry, South London and Maudsley NHS Trust London, Ladywell Unit, University Hospital Lewisham, London SE13 6LH

Rosie Illingworth, Lecturer in Communication, Medical Education Unit, University of Manchester, Rusholme Health Centre, Walmer Street, Manchester M14 5NP

Cornelius Katona, Dean, Royal College of Psychiatrists, 1998–2003; Dean, Kent Institute of Medicine and Health Sciences, University of Kent, Canterbury CT2 7PD

Brian Lunn, Senior Lecturer, School of Neurology, Neurobiology and Psychiatry, University of Newcastle, Royal Victoria Infirmary, Queen Victoria Road, Newcastle upon Tyne NE1 4LP

Pavan Mallikarjun, Senior House Officer, All Birmingham Rotation Training Scheme, Birmingham B15 2QZ

Albert Michael, Consultant Psychiatrist, West Suffolk Hospital, Bury St Edmunds IP33 2QZ; Director, Cambridge MRCPsych Course, Fulbourn Hospital, Cambridge CB1 5EF

Rory O'Shea, Specialist Registrar, Department of Psychiatry, Park House, Nursery Road, Huntingdon PE29 3RJ

Abdul Rahim Patel, Consultant in Old Age Psychiatry, Queen Elizabeth Psychiatric Hospital, Mindelsohn Way, Edgbaston, Birmingham B15 2QZ

Iain Pryde, Specialist Registrar, Old Age and General Adult Psychiatry, MHOA Team B, 59 Cordwell Road, Lewisham, London SE13 5QY

Ranga Rao, Consultant Psychiatrist/Senior Lecturer, GKT MRCPsych Course Organiser, South London and Maudsley NHS Trust, Ladywell Unit, University Hospital Lewisham, London SE13 6LW

Amrit Sachar, Specialist Registrar, Adult Psychiatry, Scutari, St Thomas' Hospital, Lambeth Palace Road, London SE1 7EH

Stephen Tyrer, former Chief Examiner, Royal College of Psychiatrists, 1998–2001; Senior Clinical Lecturer, University of Newcastle, Consultant Psychiatrist in Neurorehabilitation and Pain, Royal Victoria Infirmary, Newcastle upon Tyne NE1 4LP

Hugh Williams, Consultant Psychiatrist, Substance Misuse Service, South Downs Health NHS Trust, 26 Ditchling Road, Brighton, East Sussex BN1 4SF; Honorary Senior Lecturer, Department of Addictive Behaviour, St George's Hospital Medical School, London SW17 ORE

Stephanie Young, Specialist Registrar, General Adult Psychiatry, Southbrook Road Mental Health Advice Centre, 1 Southbrook Road, London SE12 8LH

Foreword

The Objective Structured Clinical Examination (OSCE) was introduced into Part I of the Membership examination of the Royal College of Psychiatrists (MRCPsych) in spring 2003. It was the most important single innovation in a raft of changes aimed at making the MRCPsych fairer, more valid and more reliable. It is ironic that, since OSCEs have for the past few years been part of undergraduate medical examinations in the UK and in other countries, many MRCPsych candidates will be more familiar with them than their educational supervisors, tutors and even perhaps their MRCPsych course organisers. Cold comfort perhaps for new recruits to psychiatry!

It might be argued that it would have been less bother and expense for candidates, for examiners and for the College to have stuck with older, tried and tested forms of examination. They worked well enough for me, so why not for today's trainees? It has to be admitted that part of the justification for OSCEs is that they are in fashion. This, though, is only a small part of the argument. Apart from anything else, OSCEs are hardly new – they have been in use in medical education for more than 20 years and are now increasingly used in the UK and across the world in specialist as well as undergraduate medical examinations. They can simulate a wide range of clinical situations and allow an individual candidate's competence to be assessed over a relatively broad clinical arena. In particular, they allow the rigorous assessment of a candidate's performance in important areas of clinical competence in psychiatry (such as communicating diagnosis, treatment or bad news to patients or relatives and discussing a complex formulation with other members of the clinical team) that are otherwise almost impossible to assess. They also reduce the 'luck of the draw' element inherent in using real patients and have been shown to mirror clinical practice better than written simulations.

I am proud, as chair of the working group that oversaw the implementation of the recent changes to the MRCPsych, that the OSCE has successfully been introduced. We now need to ensure that candidates have the best possible preparation for this element of the MRCPsych. Dr Rao and his colleagues are to be congratulated for producing a scholarly yet readable guide, which goes a long way to meeting that need. It will be a substantial help to candidates preparing for psychiatric OSCEs – and to their teachers.

Professor Cornelius Katona
Dean, Royal College of Psychiatrists, 1998–2003

Abbreviations

A&E	accident and emergency
CPN	community psychiatric nurse
CPR	cardiopulmonary resuscitation
CT	computerised tomography
ECT	electroconvulsive therapy
GMC	General Medical Council
GP	general practitioner
MRCPsych	Membership examination of the Royal College of Psychiatrists
MRI	magnetic resonance imaging
NHS	National Health Service
OSCE	Objective Structured Clinical Examination
PLAB	Professional and Linguistic Assessment Board

Introduction

Ranga Rao

This book is intended to be a guide for those who are taking the Objective Structured Clinical Examination (OSCE) component of Part I of the Membership examination of the Royal College of Psychiatrists. However, it will also be helpful for any postgraduate examination in psychiatry where an OSCE format is used, as in the assessment of basic training of the Royal Australian and New Zealand College of Psychiatrists. Contributions have been invited from a wide range of clinicians who have expertise in the area and reflect most of the dimensions of OSCEs. The Royal College of Psychiatrists introduced the OSCE format of examination in spring 2003. Before the publication of this book, there will have been at least two rounds of examinations conducted by the College. This should be generating useful information about the conduct of the examination. In the meantime, the aims, format and content of the OSCE is explained on the College website, at www.rcpsych.ac.uk/traindev/exams/regulation/osce1.htm.

The book is divided into two parts, and is accompanied by a CD–ROM. I hope that all three elements will be of assistance in preparing you to pass Part I of the College Membership examination in its new format.

Part I

Part I is focused on general aspects of the OSCE. Chapter 1, on the theoretical context of the OSCE, is intended to give you a brief background. Chapter 2 is by Dr Stephen Tyrer, the former Chief Examiner of the Royal College of Psychiatrists; it explains the development of OSCEs from the College perspective. In Chapter 3, Brian Lunn describes how OSCEs are generated and the 'stations' (a booth generally occupied by an actor playing the part of a patient) for the examination created. You might consider how you would create some of your own stations after reading this chapter. As OSCEs primarily involve communication and interviewing skills, Chapter 4, by Linda Gask and Rosie Illingworth, covers these in some detail. In Chapter 5, Peter Bowie gives you some helpful tips and techniques to get through this component of the Membership examination.

While all of the above chapters should prove a useful source of information for consultant trainers as well, the last chapter in Part I, by Abdul Rahim Patel and Pavan Mallikarjun, is more directed at educational supervisors, and covers training issues. Trainees may also wish to be aware of the contents of this chapter to get an idea of what to expect from consultant trainers and use this during supervision.

Part II

Part II of the book is entirely devoted to specific scenarios you are likely to come across in the OSCE. The aim is not to present every possible scenario, which would not have been possible in a book of reasonable length. Instead, the focus has been on the main diagnostic entities you might come across. Aspects of technique are emphasised throughout; you will clearly also be expected to have the required theoretical knowledge. Within each chapter the constructs have been devised in such a way that they appear realistic and can be covered within 7 minutes – the designated time in the OSCE to be spent at each station. It is important to remember that the marking of the OSCE is very much related to the dimensions of the construct. The 'Suggested approach' sections within each chapter are provided to give you some prompts for questions in each area. You should be able to pick up the common thread and develop your own technique for confronting any particular station. For example, the general approach for explaining diagnosis and prognosis in schizophrenia is obviously applicable to other illnesses as well.

Throughout the whole book, aspects of communication are emphasised, but Chapter 13, on stations that predominantly test candidates' communication skills, is particularly relevant in this regard. The communication of results of biological investigations is covered in Chapter 14. The most difficult thing to put down on paper is how to go about examining a patient; this is something that you ideally need to see rather than read in a book. Anish Bahra has translated this formidable task into the chapter on neurological examination, and you will see that the style and layout of this chapter is different from the others.

Essentially, going through the whole book should prepare you for most of the stations you are likely to encounter, but you may of course tailor your use to suit your specific needs.

CD–ROM

On the CD–ROM that accompanies this book we have included a number of sample OSCE scenarios for you to watch; these focus on aspects of communication and how these may influence the conduct of your interview – and potentially your success in the examination. You will gain most benefit if you follow the instructions and use the scenarios as interactively as possible, rather than passively watching them all the way through in one sitting. Each clip is designed to illustrate a different set of skills, hence I would urge you to work through them all to explore different aspects of each task in detail. In some scenarios you might see how the outcome is different because a particular interview style has been adopted.

Acknowledgements

I am indebted to Professor Femi Oyebode, Chief Examiner, Royal College of Psychiatrists, for his encouragement, support and suggestions from inception to the completion of the typescript. I am also grateful to Stephen Antao, my personal assistant, for all the secretarial help with the typescript, while keeping on top of the enormous load of clinical work. Finally, I would like to acknowledge the enthusiasm, commitment and dedication of my colleague assistant course organisers/specialist registrars Dr Amrit Sachar, Dr Amanda Hukin, Dr Iain Pryde and Dr Stephanie Young, who have undertaken the challenging task of translating the idea of the CD–ROM into reality.

Part I
Background and general approaches

CHAPTER 1

OSCEs: the theoretical background

Ranga Rao

In medical education, the traditional and well-established method of evaluating a candidate's performance in an examination has been the 'long case', in which the candidate is required to assess a patient comprehensively and present the findings to examiners. This process involves a complex interplay of factors, is difficult to standardise and is, to a large extent, subjective. In view of this, changes to the examination system have been introduced in an attempt to increase its objectivity, and to make the outcome of the examination more dependent on the candidate's performance. The OSCE is an attempt in this direction.

The introduction of OSCEs

Harden & Gleeson (1979) were the first to describe an OSCE, as a 'timed examination in which medical students interact with a series of simulated patients, in stations that may involve history taking, physical examination, counselling or patient management'. Because of their feasibility, OSCEs have become widespread for performance-based assessment, particularly in undergraduate examinations, for which they are now used in most medical schools in London, for example. Their use was pioneered by the Royal London and St Bartholomew's Hospital. Several of the medical Royal Colleges have introduced an OSCE component into their postgraduate Membership examinations. In keeping with this, the Royal College of Psychiatrists introduced an OSCE into Part I of its Membership examination in spring 2003.

Advantages and disadvantages

The advantages and disadvantages of OSCEs are summarised in Box 1.1. Compared with a traditional long case, an OSCE has the advantage of allowing different students to be presented with a similar task, as the variability of patient-related factors is reduced. With training, actors

---

Box 1.1 Advantages and disadvantages of Objective Structured Clinical Examinations

Advantages
• Simulations of real-life situations
• Close to reality
• Controlled and safe
• Feedback is available from the actors (simulators)
• Ready availability when required
• Stations can be tailored to the level of skill to be assessed
• Scenarios that are distressing to real patients can be simulated
• The patient variable in examination is uniform across trainees.

Disadvantages
• Idealised 'textbook' scenarios may not mimic real-life situations
• Short stations may not allow the assessment of complex skills
• Cost
• Training issues in setting up the stations.

From Wallace *et al* (2002), with permission.

---

can simulate many real-life situations and, unlike with real patients, one need not be worried about the effect of repeated questioning on their mental state – hence, in that sense, they are reasonably controlled and safe. Simulated patients are readily available and can be trained to portray a patient repeatedly and consistently.

The disadvantages of OSCEs are mainly to do with the fact that short stations do not always allow the proper assessment of complex skills. Even though OSCEs are good at assessing specific tasks, skills such as complex reasoning may not be accurately assessed. Cost is also an important factor and there are enormous training issues in setting up the stations. Further, there may be a sense of artificiality, as the idealised textbook scenarios may not exactly mimic real-life situations.

The uses of OSCEs

The OSCE format with simulated patients is used in a range of settings (Wallace *et al*, 2002) (see Box 1.2).

Communication skills are an essential element to the doctor–patient relationship and these can be assessed as the simulated patients can provide feedback on important interview skills such as empathy. Hodges *et al* (1996) assessed this and concluded that communication OSCE stations can be created with acceptable reliability; typical cases address communication skills beyond simple history-taking.

> **Box 1.2** Uses of the OSCE format
>
> - Teaching communication skills
> - Teaching clinical skills
> - Monitoring the performance of doctors
> - Clinical examinations.
>
> From Wallace *et al* (2002), with permission.

Monitoring doctors' performance is another area where OSCEs have been used and this was examined in a primary-care setting in The Netherlands (Rethans & van Boven, 1987). Data were collected about general practitioners' performance by testing their skill in managing urinary tract infections according to a consensus guideline. The same group (Rethans *et al*, 1991) replicated this for other clinical problems such as headache, diarrhoea and shoulder pain, and found that general practitioners' performance on the whole was shown to be an accurate reflection of their actual practice.

Another study in primary care (McClure *et al*, 1985) assessed the family physician's ability to collect diagnostic information and formulate a management plan. They used trained patients with uncomplicated rheumatic disease and found that even though most physicians neglected areas such as psychosocial impact and mental health issues, they made an adequate assessment and developed a coherent care plan.

Norman *et al* (1982) studied clinical skills assessment using a sample of ten residents and compared their performance on four real patients with chronic stable conditions and four simulated patients who were trained to present the same problems. They reported no significant differences in the number of questions asked in the history-taking, findings from the physical examination, diagnosis or investigations proposed. Residents correctly identified 67% of the patients as real or simulated.

Besides their use in teaching, in improving communication skills and in monitoring doctors' performance, much of the literature has focused on the use of OSCEs in formal examinations of students' clinical skills. These are discussed in the subsequent sections.

Validity and reliability of OSCEs

Considering that OSCEs are used in a wide range of settings, it is worth examining the issues of their reliability and validity. Generally, validity refers to accuracy and reliability to consistency of performance.

In medical education we aim to assess competence; this would amount to construct validity, while correlation with the results of other forms of assessment would represent concurrent validity. These aspects were assessed by Hodges *et al* (1998), who attempted to demonstrate construct validity by comparing the performance of residents and medical students. They also assessed concurrent validity by asking tutors responsible for students to rate them on interviewing skills. The tutors were generally able to predict these ratings, which correlated with the OSCE marks. Content validity asks how real the simulations by actors were – and, indirectly, how representative the sample was of the general patient population. This aspect was also assessed in the same study by asking residents how real these simulations were: 80% described the scenarios as real or very real.

Hodges *et al* (1999) also assessed the relationship between results on a binary ('yes' or 'no') content checklist and levels of competence as measured by the OSCE. Their sample included clinical clerks, family practice residents and family physicians, who participated in two 15-minute standardised patient interviews. Their results indicated that on global scales (judgements made in a particular domain), experienced clinicians scored significantly more than residents and clerks, but on the checklist, the latter scored better than experienced clinicians. They concluded that binary checklists may not be a valid assessment of clinical competence. This factor may be important in the context of postgraduate examinations.

As mentioned above, Hodges *et al* (1996) evaluated communication skills in the context of the OSCE format and commented that communication OSCE stations can be created with acceptable reliability but cautioned against their generalisability. Martin & Jolly (2002) assessed the ability of an OSCE taken at the end of the first clinical year to predict later performance in clinical examinations. They studied the OSCE performance of two consecutive cohorts of third-year medical undergraduates and compared this with their performance in the clinical examination in years four and five. The early OSCE assessments strongly predicted later clinical performance.

It could be argued that there would be a differential response to real and simulated patients. This was investigated by Sanson-Fisher & Poole (1980), who assessed this using a group of second-year medical students. They did not find any significant differences in levels of empathy between students' interactions with genuine or simulated patients. In fact, the students were unable to discriminate between the two groups of patients.

Wood *et al* (1999) attempted to design a clinical examination of high content validity for assessing pre-registration house officers from the St Bartholomew's and Royal London School of Medicine in London. An OSCE was used as the main outcome measure. The authors concluded that the OSCE format can be used to provide 'real-life scenarios'.

A different type of study, from the University of Kentucky College of Medicine (Valentino et al, 1998), was conducted on the subject of the reliability of OSCEs. This attempted to measure the agreement among faculty members about the importance of items on a checklist used to grade candidates at each OSCE station. The results strongly suggested that a group of faculty members is able to enhance the reliability of OSCE grading relative to what can be achieved by one person.

From the foregoing, it appears that OSCEs generally do seem to have acceptable reliability and validity; however, much of the work appears to have been with undergraduates.

The fact that some stations are repeated in the OSCE setting raises questions about security. This issue was examined by Niehaus et al (1996) with a group of medical students in a study where OSCE stations were repeated in three or four rotations within a single academic year. They found no consistent evidence that students scored increasingly higher on the stations that were repeated, and concluded that station repetition did not risk a trend towards increasing scores. The opportunity for a further study (Wilkinson et al, 2003) arose when a third of the students were inadvertently given station names before their OSCE. There was no significant difference in the overall marks of the students who had this advantage and those who did not.

In spite of the general optimism about the use of OSCEs, there are some reservations as to whether they are the solution to all problems. While assessing medical students' examinations, Konje et al (2001) commented on the discriminatory value of OSCEs in assessing the clinical competence of medical students. They found that only 11% of the variability in their competence could be explained by their performance on OSCEs and they cautioned against completely replacing clinical examinations with OSCEs.

OSCEs and psychiatry

Even though OSCEs have been evaluated in many other disciplines in medicine, there are few papers concerning their use in psychiatry. The first of these was from Nigeria, by Famuyiwa et al (1991), who investigated whether this format of examination was effective and valid. They compared the OSCE scores of 123 students with criterion-based reference scores on multiple-choice questions and found that multiple-choice marks correlated significantly with OSCE ratings.

Hodges and colleagues at the University of Toronto have since contributed significantly to this area. In 1997 they evaluated the feasibility, reliability and validity of the OSCE for psychiatric clinical clerks. They concluded that a psychiatric OSCE is feasible for assessing complex psychiatric skills. They stressed the importance of a range of issues, particularly the training of simulated patients, and commented on the costs of the examinations as well (Hodges et al, 1997). In a subsequent paper (Hodges et al, 1998) they examined the validity of an OSCE in psychiatry by comparing the performance of residents and clerks (see above). They found evidence for both construct and concurrent validity, and went on to suggest that a psychiatric OSCE can be a valid assessment of a clerk's clinical competence. In a further study (Hodges et al, 1999) they reported that 80% of residents who took the clerkship examination agreed that simulations were realistic and reflected situations that psychiatric residents would come across.

In another report, the same group (Hanson et al, 1998) reported on the successful integration of child psychiatry into a psychiatric clerkship OSCE. They developed OSCE stations for four common child psychiatric conditions and reported on their reliability as well as the financial cost of their development. In a different type of study, Coyle et al (1998) examined the use of substituting standardised patients in psychotherapy teaching. They used experienced mental health counsellors as standardised patients and felt that this enhanced the realism of the situation.

As in other areas, the use of OSCEs in psychiatry has been limited but has generally supported its feasibility.

Conclusions

On the whole, the literature on OSCEs suggests that it is possible to create OSCE stations with a fair degree of reliability and validity for use in different settings. With regard to the marking sheets, it appears that global ratings rather than checklists are a better method of assessment in postgraduate examinations. Training of the role-payers has been generally emphasised as a way of enhancing validity and this issue assumes more importance when complex psychiatric scenarios are potrayed. Much of the work done in this area has been in undergraduate education and it remains to be seen whether it can endure the same rigour of evaluation in postgraduate education.

At a time when there appears to be an emerging consensus about their utility, an interesting study (Wass et al, 2001) compared the long case with the OSCE format of assessment. The authors concluded that long cases, in terms of reliability, are 'no worse and no better than OSCEs in assessing clinical competence'.

Thus it would seem that what matters is not the format in which one is examined but how standardised the examination is. There is increasing evidence to support the fact that it would be easier to develop OSCEs further as a way of ensuring the objectivity and fairness that trainees deserve.

References

Coyle, B., Miller, M. & McGowen, K. R. (1998) Using standardized patients to teach and learn psychotherapy. *Academic Medicine*, **73**, 591–592.

Famuyiwa, O. O., Zachariah, M. P. & Ilechukwu, S. T. C. (1991) The objective structured clinical examination in undergraduate psychiatry. *Medical Education*, **25**, 45–50.

Hanson, M., Hodges, B., McNaughton, N., *et al* (1998) The integration of child psychiatry into a psychiatry clerkship OSCE. *Canadian Journal of Psychiatry*, **43**, 614–618.

Harden, R. M. & Gleeson, F. A. (1979) Assessment of clinical competence using an objective structured clinical examination (OSCE). *Medical Education*, **13**, 41–54.

Hodges, B., Turnbull, J., Cohen, R., *et al* (1996) Evaluating communication skills in the OSCE format: reliability and generalizability. *Medical Education*, **30**, 38–43.

Hodges, B., Regehr, G., Hanson, M., *et al* (1997) An objective structured clinical examination for evaluating psychiatric clinical clerks. *Academic Medicine*, **72**, 715–721.

Hodges, B., Regehr, G., Hanson, M., *et al* (1998) Validation of an objective structured clinical examination in psychiatry. *Academic Medicine*, **73**, 910–912.

Hodges, B., Regehr, G., McNaughton, N., *et al* (1999) OSCE checklists do not capture increasing levels of expertise. *Academic Medicine*, **74**, 1129–1134.

Konje, C., Abrams, K. R. & Taylor, J. (2001) How discriminatory is the objective structured clinical examination (OSCE) in the assessment of clinical competence of medical students? *Journal of Obstetrics and Gynaecology*, **21**, 223–227.

Martin, I. G. & Jolly, B. (2002) Predictive validity and estimated cut score of an objective structured clinical examination (OSCE) used as an assessment of clinical skills at the end of the first clinical year. *Medical Education*, **36**, 418–425.

McClure, C. L., Gall, E., Meredith, K. E., *et al* (1985) Assessing clinical judgement with standardized patients. *Journal of Family Practice*, **20**, 457–464.

Niehaus, A. H., DaRosa, D. A., Markwell, S. J., *et al* (1996) Is test security a concern when OSCE stations are repeated across clerkship rotations? *Academic Medicine*, **71**, 287–289.

Norman, G. R., Tugwell, P. & Feightner, J. W. (1982) A comparison of resident performance on real and simulated patients. *Journal of Medical Education*, **27**, 708–715.

Rethans, J. J. & van Boven, C. P. (1987) Simulated patients in general practice: a different look at the consultation. *British Medical Journal*, **294**, 809–812.

Rethans, J. J., Sturmans, F., Drop, R., *et al* (1991) Assessment of the performance of general practitioners by the use of standardized (simulated) patients. *British Journal of General Practice*, **41**, 97–99.

Sanson-Fisher, R. W. & Poole, A. D. (1980) Simulated patients and the assessment of medical students' interpersonal skills. *Medical Education*, **14**, 249–253.

Valentino, J., Donnelly, M. B., Sloan, D. A., *et al* (1998) The reliability of six faculty members in identifying important OSCE items. *Academic Medicine*, **73**, 204–205.

Wallace, J., Rao, R. & Haslam, R. (2002) Simulated patients and objective structured clinical examinations: review of their use in medical education. *Advances in Psychiatric Treatment*, **8**, 342–350.

Wass, V., Jones, R. & Van der Vleuten, C. (2001) Standardized or real patients to test clinical competence? The long case revisited. *Medical Education*, **35**, 321–325.

Wilkinson, T. J., Fontaine, S. & Egan, T. (2003) Was a breach of examination security unfair in an objective structured clinical examination. *Medical Teaching*, **25**, 42–46.

Wood, D., Roberts, T., Bradley, P., *et al* (1999) 'Hello, my name is Gabriel, I am the house officer, may I examine you?' or the Objective Santa Christmas Examination (OSCE). *Medical Education*, **33**, 915–919.

CHAPTER 2

Development of the OSCE: a College perspective

Stephen Tyrer

Following the inquiry into the Bristol paediatric heart surgeons' culpability regarding their poor performance, the need to determine, monitor and regulate the proficiency of doctors became a pressing concern (Klein, 1998). Further action was required by the state and the assessment of the clinical competence of doctors became imperative. It was no coincidence that one year after the Bristol inquiry, the government started the process of what is now called clinical governance (NHS Executive, 1999). The principal tenet of clinical governance is the delivery of high-quality health care. A recent paper, of which the current Chief Medical Officer was a co-author, emphasised what this means in any organisation within the NHS. Each organisation should be 'accountable for continually improving the quality of its services and safeguarding high standards of care by creating an environment in which excellence in clinical care will flourish' (Halligan & Donaldson, 1999).

In order to assure high quality of clinical care, practitioners need to be capable in what they do. The Royal Colleges in the UK have a key role in determining what is a sufficient level of competence in each medical discipline. Only those doctors who have attained an acceptable degree of clinical competence in their specialty should be able to practise in a senior capacity.

Examination of a specialist area in medical knowledge should include the following:

- knowledge of the basic sciences and clinical topics
- comprehension of the clinical problems
- communication skills
- analysis of factual and clinical knowledge
- evaluation of this material
- synthesis of this information
- application of this knowledge and information.

The Membership examination

The Royal College of Psychiatrists developed its Membership examination, customarily abbreviated to the MRCPsych, almost immediately after the College was founded in 1971. The prime aim of the examination was, and still is, to set a standard that determines whether candidates are suitable to progress to higher professional training at a specialist registrar level. In addition, possession of the qualification is considered to be an indicator of professional competence in the clinical practice of psychiatry.

The first MRCPsych examinations were designed to test factual knowledge of both the sciences basic to psychiatry and the fundamentals of history-taking and mental state examination, in addition to clinical skills. The examination has always been in two parts. Part I is taken after one year of specialist training in psychiatry and the written part of this examination has always been in multiple-choice format. This is followed by a clinical examination (which has been in the form of an Observed Structured Clinical Examination (OSCE) since 2003). Both parts of the examination need to be passed concurrently in order for the candidate to succeed.

Possession of Part I of the Membership examination enables the candidate to advance to training in the sub-specialties before taking Part II after a further 18 months of training (this used to be 2 years).

The aim of Part I is to select those candidates who have reached a sufficient standard to progress to the next stage of instruction. In effect, Part I is a screening test that ensures that only candidates who have achieved a certain level of expertise can go on to higher training. The examination also provides a test for both candidates and clinical tutors to assess whether further training is likely to result in a subsequent pass mark in the Part II examination.

The multiple-choice paper of Part I is able to test knowledge but there is no opportunity in this type of examination for clinical reasoning and evaluation to take place. Examination of the last six elements in the list above cannot be assessed through this format. These skills need to be tested in the Part I clinical examination. Until spring 2003, the candidate had to take a history and mental state examination from a patient within 1 hour and present the case in a 30-minute interview with the examiners. This format, the 'long case', has now been replaced by the OSCE. Why has this change been made?

The assessment of clinical competence

Clinical examination of a real patient in an examination is a test of the ability of the candidate to be able to communicate effectively with a patient and provide a supportive environment in which the patient is able to confide his or her difficulties to the doctor. This format of examination also permits assessment of the ability of the candidate to evaluate, synthesise and summarise clinical information in an acceptable form. However, there are considerable limitations in this procedure in an examination which permits entry to higher training.

Real patients selected for any clinical examination are bound to vary considerably in the degree of difficulty their case presents. The patient may be difficult to communicate with as a result, for example, of prolixity, the presentation of much irrelevant information, a strong regional accent or speech defects. These haphazard factors may adversely affect the capacity of the candidate to take an adequate history.

The long case was supposed to test the ability of the candidate to communicate with patients. However, in Part I of the MRCPsych examination the interview with the patient was not observed by the examiners and this skill could be observed only indirectly. Candidates were tested on the information they obtained from the patient and on their ability to organise this material successfully. Although the patient was invited by the candidate into the room with the examiners and asked to carry out a separate clinical test, this part of the examination lasted for only 10 minutes. None of the information from the previous hour's interview was available to the examiners and could not be tested, except in an artificial situation.

It has been shown that the relationship between the skill of interviewing a patient and the ability to present to examiners facts resulting from the interview is not close. Wass & Jolly (2001) found that the correlation between these two skills was low, at between 0.33 and 0.38, depending on how the assessment was marked. Furthermore, in that same study, direct observation of the history-taking procedure contributed as much again to overall performance as the presentation of the case.

The ratings by the examiners of communication skills in the history-taking component and presentation performance contributed significantly and independently to a rating of clinical competence. This suggests that these two different skills measured separate parameters of clinical proficiency. In practice, in an examination involving a long case, although there are clearly advantages in rating the interviews with the patient and the session with the examiners separately, the logistics and time implications for the examiners in assessing such material is impractical in the time available. In addition, it has been shown that the reliability of the assessment of clinical competency from a single patient case is low and it has been estimated that 10 such long cases would be required in an examination to assess clinical competence reliably (Wass et al, 2001). The main reason for this is because of patient variability (sometimes known as case specificity). Case specificity means that performance with one patient-related problem does not reliably predict performance with subsequent problems (Norman *et al*, 1985). It is not a surprise that assessment of clinical ability in general in patients with different diagnoses cannot be made on the basis of performance on a single case.

Because of concerns about both Part I and Part II of the Membership examination, the advice of a medical educationalist was sought in 1998. The educationalist concerned, Helen Mulholland, recommended a number of alterations, the reasons for which have been described elsewhere (Katona *et al*, 2000; Tyrer & Oyebode, 2004). She was particularly concerned about the wide case specificity in the Part I examination and after an options appraisal a decision was made to discontinue the long case from the Part I examination and replace this with a more reliable examination of clinical skills. The OSCE was recommended as the preferred format.

Reasons for choosing the OSCE

The main reason for selecting the OSCE format was to assess the clinical performance of candidates over a sufficient range of patient problems. The advantage of an OSCE is that a circuit of stations, normally numbering between 10 and 16, enables each candidate to be tested on as many different scenarios as there are stations. Each OSCE station tests a specific skill or technique. Although it is necessary to have 'standardised' (i.e. simulated) patients in most stations, and these are obviously different from real patients, the advantage is that they are able to act out identical scenarios consistently for each candidate who appears before them. In addition, examiners can evaluate directly the communication skills of the candidates as well as their ability to organise a sequence of clinical questions in a coherent form. The examiner is therefore better able to assess communication skills than in a long case .

The evidence that OSCEs assess clinical skills independently of medical facts has recently been demonstrated inadvertently in an assessment of medical undergraduates in New Zealand (Wilkinson *et al*, 2003*a*). One-third of the undergraduates being assessed on an OSCE were informed accidentally of the nature of the stations that were going to be used. Despite the consequent opportunity to revise before the examination, the group that was forewarned performed no better than the other two groups, with not even a trend towards higher scores.

Smee (2003) showed that OSCEs are effective as a screen for the presence or absence of sufficient clinical skills. The assessment of these abilities at an early stage of training is important in a discipline such as psychiatry, which relies on skills of communication with patients

17

(Broquet, 2002). The majority of candidates who have achieved a sufficient standard in the theoretical grounding of psychiatry and who have had sufficient exposure to the assessment of patients should pass Part I of the Membership examination. In an examination of this type it is not necessary to distinguish between the borderline pass and the excellent candidate – all are considered sufficiently competent to progress to the next stage. The examination acts, therefore, as a tool to screen out those candidates who are not yet considered to be sufficiently clinically competent to proceed to higher training.

There is, however, some evidence that OSCEs are not effective at the assessment of higher degrees of ability, although this does depend on the method of rating (Hodges *et al*, 1999).

Alternative formats

Other assessment measures were considered as a way of assessing clinical competence at the end of Part I training. These included:

- extending the long case and having the examiners observe the complete interaction between the candidate and the patient
- assessing the candidates on three or four short cases
- assessing the candidates on a series of patient vignettes, with probes and questions from the examiners.

An in-depth assessment of a long case has been proposed, the Objective Structured Long Examination Record (OSLER) (Gleeson, 1994). This procedure involves direct observation of the candidate interacting with the patient. The importance of this assessment in a discipline such as psychiatry is self-evident and this technique has been used with success in evaluating undergraduates in psychiatry (Price & Byrne, 1994). However, to provide a valid assessment of ability in this sphere patients with a variety of different diagnoses need to be interviewed. The time and complexity involved in arranging an examination of this nature render it impractical for the MRCPsych Part I examination.

The other options were also discarded because of the acknowledged greater utility and reliability of the OSCE (Famuyiwa *et al*, 1991; Sloan *et al*, 1996; Hodges *et al*, 1997). Although the proposal for a series of structured patient management problems has a number of advantages, it was felt that these same skills could be adequately tested at this level of training within an OSCE format.

Development of the OSCE

Whenever a modification to the MRCPsych examination is formally proposed, a working party is constituted to examine the content and design of the new component. An OSCE working party was therefore constituted with the present Chief Examiner, Professor Femi Oyebode, appointed as its chairman. It was agreed that a pilot OSCE should be set up to determine its feasibility, that a scoring system be developed for it and that further pilot examinations should then be arranged to refine the process. In all, three pilot examinations were held, in London and Leeds.

It was agreed early that simulated patients would be used in the OSCE, at least in the first few examinations. The main reason for this was to ensure standardisation of the patient material. In the event, the number of actors and actresses required for the examination has not proved a problem and the ability of these individuals to convey psychiatric symptoms has been extremely good. Most candidates are quite unable to determine whether they are seeing a real patient or an actor.

The selection of the stations on the first OSCE was 'blueprinted' according to the curriculum (see Chapter 3). Blueprinting refers to a process in which the core items in a curriculum of knowledge are determined and these abilities are assessed by a particular examination in the skill or competency concerned.

It was proposed that 12 stations be selected in the OSCE, as this number had been found to be practical and yet test the candidate in a sufficient number of areas to appraise clinical skills adequately. It was agreed that the majority of the stations should be concerned with the assessment of standardised patients or relatives and only two or three stations should be used for the assessment of physical signs, in a model.

It was helpful when selecting stations for use in the pilot OSCEs to ask the following questions:

- Are the patient problems relevant and important to core items in the curriculum?
- Have a sufficient number of experts from all disciplines reviewed the stations and determined these to be important in the assessment of core psychiatric skills?
- Do the stations assess skills that have been taught?

The stations

All OSCE stations have four components: a construct; instructions to candidates; objectives; and instructions to simulated patients.

Construct

The construct describes the setting of the station and what the candidate is aiming to achieve in the task. For example, in a station concerned with explaining to an anxious relative the treatment options, course and prognosis of a young man with obsessive–compulsive disorder (OCD) the aims would include explanation of the principles of treatment and the uncertain prognosis at this stage in the illness. The need for careful explanation in lay language would be an essential skill in this station.

Instructions to candidates

The instructions to the candidates in a station of this nature would be along the lines of the following:

'Mr James Robson is a 22-year-old man whom you have seen in your out-patient clinic; he has checking rituals associated with marked worries of contamination. The most likely diagnosis is obsessive–compulsive disorder. You are asked to see Mr Robson's mother to explain the nature of this illness, to indicate treatments that may be used and to describe the prognosis.'

Objectives

The objectives that the candidate has to achieve are tasks selected according to the information indicated in the construct. Tasks are chosen that are appropriate to the level of training for a Part I candidate and that can be observed accurately by the examiner. Thus, explanation to a relative of the non-psychotic nature of OCD and the technique of response prevention would comprise two tasks that would be rated by the examiner.

The tasks are marked according to the perceived ability of the candidate to address the issues involved. The marking is done by a single examiner at the station, who acknowledges the candidate only at the beginning and end of the OSCE. The candidate should address all discourse to the simulated patient or relative concerned.

The sections to be scored by the examiner are not made according to a pre-arranged list. On the contrary, a large proportion of the marks awarded is allocated according to the ability of the candidate to communicate the information required appropriately to the relative or patient. The facility to explain the treatment options and further explanation of the prognosis in the condition would also be scored separately. Each item is rated on a scale from A to F, where F indicates a very severe fail, and D and E indicate different degrees of failure. A global rating of performance is made but is not at present used in an individual's assessment.

Instructions to simulated patients

The actors and actresses simulating patients need to be informed in detail about the scenario in which they are partaking. They are given details of the psychiatric problem and its degree of severity. This includes a short history of the person and the development of symptoms. Each simulated patient is also given a summary of the issues that might be considered by the candidate. Thus, in the case described this might include:

- what obsessive–compulsive neurosis is
- what causes it
- whether it is hereditary
- what treatments are available
- whether psychological treatments work
- what the treatments involve
- whether the drug treatments are wholly safe.

Setting standards

The criteria for passing or failing an OSCE need to be carefully determined. It is educationally sound that when important pass–fail decisions are being made the assessment should be 'criterion referenced'. This means that the examiners should determine what the standards are in each clinical station, and not simply rely on total scores on checklists of objectives (Hodges *et al*, 1999; Wilkinson *et al*, 2003*b*). Trainees should be assessed relative to performance standards rather than to each other or to a reference group.

A number of studies have shown that pass–fail decisions are made more appropriately by examiners deciding on the pass mark for each station according to the performance of borderline candidates (Smee & Blackmore, 2001; Humphrey-Murto & MacFadyen, 2002). In the traditional OSCE approach, originally described by Angoff (1971), judges decide beforehand on what a borderline candidate is likely to achieve in the task concerned. This, however, does not take into account the performance of the candidates at the time of carrying out the task. When this is assessed, the results obtained have face validity and this has been confirmed by research examining the relationship of such assessments with other measures of clinical competence (Wilkinson *et al*, 2001).

Conclusions

The development of an OSCE takes a good deal of time and preparation. Actors need to be trained, the objectives of each proposed station need to be carefully designed and all stations need to be piloted before being used in any examination (Smee, 2003). Examiners need to be trained and their performance and those of the actors needs to be monitored. An OSCE is costly. Despite this, the move to the OSCE format has been regarded favourably from both an educational and practice standpoint. Students who pass a well-designed OSCE are predicted to be competent at managing common problems in general adult and old age psychiatry. Their exact place in the MRCPsych examination will need to be determined by an analysis of results, but optimism about their potential value in assessment is high.

There is considerable evidence to indicate that OSCEs are a reliable test of clinical skills (Sloan *et al*, 1996; Hodges *et al*, 1997). As with all types of examinations, it is more important, but also more difficult, to prove the validity of OSCEs in predicting ability, as it is necessary to follow up candidates for a period of time following the examination to determine outcome. Furthermore, a candidate who has failed the examination is bound to have a more restricted career than somebody who has passed. As success in the future depends on passing the examination, it becomes a self-evident truth that passing the examination is advantageous and reaps benefits.

However, analysis of an undergraduate psychiatry OSCE has shown concurrent validity with other tests of clinical competence (Hodges *et al*, 1998). Furthermore, the introduction of an OSCE in an undergraduate examination in New Zealand changed the learning behaviour of students from the pursuit of theoretical knowledge to the attainment of practical skills (Melding *et al*, 2002).

It has been shown that OSCEs do assess specific clinical skills and that these can be evaluated as effectively in a psychiatry OSCE as in a medically based discipline (Hodges *et al*, 1997; Broquet, 2002; Melding *et al*, 2002). They are likely to remain.

References

Angoff, W. H. (1971) Scales, norms and equivalent scores. In *Educational Measurement* (ed. R. L. Thorndike), pp. 508–600. Washington, DC: American Council on Education.

Broquet, K. (2002) Using an objective structured clinical examination in a psychiatry residency. *Academic Psychiatry*, **26**, 197–201.

Famuyiwa, O. O., Zachariah, M. P. & Ilechukwu, S. T. C. (1991) The objective structured clinical exam in psychiatry. *Medical Education*, **25**, 45–50.

Gleeson, F. (1994) The effect of immediate clinical feedback on clinical skills using the OSLER. In *Proceedings of the Sixth Ottawa Conference of Medical Education* (ed. R. C. A. I. Rothman), pp. 412–415. Toronto: University of Toronto Bookstore Custom Publishing.

Halligan, A. & Donaldson, L. (1999) Implementing clinical governance: turning vision into reality. *British Medical Journal*, **322**, 1413–1417.

Hodges, B., Regehr, G., Hanson, M., *et al* (1997) An objective structured clinical examination for evaluating psychiatric clinical clerks. *Academic Medicine*, **72**, 715–721.

Hodges, B., Regehr, G., Hanson, M., *et al* (1998) Validation of an objective structured clinical examination in psychiatry. *Academic Medicine*, **73**, 910–912.

Hodges, B., Regehr, G., McNaughton, N., *et al* (1999) OSCE checklists do not capture increasing levels of expertise. *Academic Medicine*, **74**, 1129–1134.

Humphrey-Murto, S. & MacFadyen, J. C. (2002) Standard setting: a comparison of case-author and modified borderline-group methods in a small-scale OSCE. *Academic Medicine*, **77**, 729–732.

Katona, C., Tyrer, S. P., & Smalls, J. (2000) Changes to the MRCPsych examinations. *Psychiatric Bulletin*, **24**, 276–278.

Klein, R. (1998) Competence, professional regulation, and the public interest. *British Medical Journal*, **316**, 1740–1742.

Melding, P., Coverdale, J. & Robinson, E. (2002) A 'fair play'? Comparison of an objective structured clinical examination of final year medical students training in psychiatry and their supervisors' appraisals. *Australasian Psychiatry*, **10**, 344–347.

NHS Executive (1999) *Clinical Governance: Quality in the new NHS.* HSC 1999/065. Leeds: NHS Executive.

Norman, G. R., Tugwell, I. P., Feightner, J. W., *et al* (1985) Knowledge and clinical problem-solving ability. *Medical Education*, **19**, 344–356.

Price, J. & Byrne, G. J. A. (1994) The direct clinical examination: an alternative method for the assessment of clinical psychiatric skills in undergraduate medical students. *Medical Education*, **28**, 120–125.

Sloan, D. A., Donnelly, M. B., Schwartz, R. W., *et al* (1996) The use of OSCE for evaluation and instruction in graduate medical education. *Journal of Surgical Research*, **63**, 225–230.

Smee, S. (2003) Skill based assessment. *British Medical Journal*, **326**, 703–706.

Smee, S. M. & Blackmore, D. E. (2001) Setting standards for an objective structured clinical examination: the borderline group method gains ground on Angoff. *Medical Education*, **35**, 1009–1010.

Tyrer, S. & Oyebode, F. (2004) Why does the MRCPsych examination need change? *British Journal of Psychiatry*, **184**, 197–199.

Wass, V. & Jolly, B. (2001) Does observation add to the validity of the long case? *Medical Education*, **35**, 729–734.

Wass, V., Jones, R. & Van der Vleuten, C. (2001) Standardised or real patients to test clinical competence? The long case revisited. *Medical Education*, **35**, 321–325.

Wilkinson, T., Newble, D. I. & Frampton, C. M. (2001) Standard setting in an observed structured clinical examination: use of global ratings of borderline performance to determine the passing score. *Medical Education*, **35**, 1043–1049.

Wilkinson, T., Fontaine, S. & Egan, T. (2003*a*) Was a breach of examination security unfair in an objective structured clinical examination? A critical incident. *Medical Teacher*, **25**, 42–46.

Wilkinson, T. J., Frampton, C. M., Thompson-Fawcett, M., *et al* (2003*b*) Objectivity in objective structured clinical examinations: checklists are no substitute for examiner commitment. *Academic Medicine*, **78**, 219–223.

CHAPTER 3

The OSCE blueprint and station development

Brian Lunn

One of the key strengths of an OSCE its the ability to test a range of core competencies for each candidate in a relatively short time. Owing to the structured nature of stations and the use of standardised patients (role-players), a marking pro forma and trained examiners, an OSCE is significantly more reliable than traditional clinical examinations, such as long cases. While reliability is relatively easy to ensure, it is also easy to be misled into thinking that this necessarily represents validity. The key to ensuring the validity of the examination is to start with the curriculum and from there establish a list of the core competencies that the examination is to assess (Royal College of Psychiatrists, 2001). From this definition of educational objectives, the examination can be generated. This chapter focuses on the structure of the examination as a whole, in terms of both planning and ensuring that an appropriate mix of stations is set. It also provides an introduction to station development

The blueprint

The 'blueprint assessment' (Dauphinee, 1994) or master plan is a useful tool that enables those setting the examination to ensure that the core competencies they set out to assess are covered. It can also be used to ensure that there is an adequate range of questions covering a suitable variety of topics.

There are certain clinical competencies that can be expected of a candidate taking Part I of the MRCPsych. The full range of these is set out by the Royal College of Psychiatrists (2001) and Box 3.1 gives a specific example related to psychopharmacology.

In the relatively short time available at each station (7 minutes for the College's Part I OSCE) it is clearly not possible to cover all aspects

Box 3.1 Clinical competencies in psychopharmacology of a candidate taking Part I of the MRCPsych

The trainee should be able:
- to appreciate and discuss the relevance of psychopharmacology to the practice of psychiatry
- to list the full range of drugs that may be used to treat psychiatric disorders, including schizophrenia (e.g. first episode, acute relapse, maintenance, refractory symptoms, special comorbidities – depression, epilepsy, cardiovascular disease – and management of side-effects) and depression (e.g. acute episode, maintenance, refractory symptoms, adjunctive treatments, depression with psychoses and special comorbidities – epilepsy and substance misuse)
- to list the full range of drugs that may be used to treat other psychiatric disorders, such as bipolar disorder, dementia, delirium, acute behavioural disturbance, alcohol and other dependencies and psychosexual disorders, together with their indications, contraindications, effects and side-effects (this will include typical and atypical antipsychotics, antidepressants, anxiolytics and mood stabilisers such as lithium, carbamazepine and sodium valproate)
- to demonstrate a working knowledge of the initial and maintenance treatment of the common psychiatric conditions listed above, as well as their management in the context of physical, other psychiatric or dependence-related comorbidity
- to obtain a drug and alcohol history in conjunction with a prescribed-drug history
- to explain to the patient the potential adverse effects of alcohol and other drugs on the course of treatment
- to understand the nature, extent and generalisability of the published evidence of efficacy of the drugs commonly used in psychiatry
- to demonstrate awareness of psychological illness, medication and social/ environmental factors that influence a patient's willingness to take medication or resistance to it, and strategies to deal with such difficulties
- to demonstrate awareness of ways of accessing data on drug effectiveness and safety.

Source: Royal College of Psychiatrists (2001, pp. 17–18)

of, for example, history-taking, but each station can focus on one aspect of history-taking and so allow a picture of a candidate's ability to be generated from a number of 'snapshots'. Table 3.1 shows some of the ways in which history-taking can be broken down – it can be subdivided into content areas derived from patient presentations, disorders or types of history, and skill areas. Unlike in traditional clinical examinations, the ability to take a corroborative history can be assessed, as can the ability to take a history where the patient presents with particular difficulties – for example, hostility or anger, areas that could never have been safely assessed previously.

Table 3.1 Ways in which history-taking can be assessed across a series of OSCE stations

Competency	Examples
Disorders	Alcohol dependence Suicidal ideation Anxiety symptoms Schizophrenia
Type of history	Corroborative history The 'difficult' patient
Skills	Focus Fluency Questioning style Empathy

This approach can be used across all the skill areas identified in the core competencies. For example, the mental state examination can be broken down into areas such as assessment of hallucinations or delusions.

It is apparent that each station will assess a number of competencies, but the temptation to assess 'as much as possible' should be resisted, as the stations need to be focused.

Blueprints are used in two ways in the MRCPsych OSCE. One is to plan each individual examination. The other defines the spread of content and skill areas to assess in the bank of developed stations. The current Part I MRCPsych OSCE is designed around 12 stations. Two blueprints are used to show, hypothetically but station by station, skill areas (Table 3.2) and content areas (Table 3.3). The two tables refer to the same circuit.

It can be seen from these hypothetical examples that each station can assess candidates' abilities across a number of domains. For example, station 2 can assess a candidate's ability to elicit from a patient with schizophrenia any delusional ideas, with a view to establishing the risk that the patient poses to others. This can then be tied to the next station, where candidates communicate their findings to the on-call consultant and discuss what they feel is the risk posed. In these examples the patient with schizophrenia would be played by a trained actor and the examiner would play the role of the on-call consultant.

The sorts of questions that need to be asked by those setting the examination are:

- Does the examination assess an appropriate mix of competencies?
- Do these competencies tally with the curriculum?
- Is the range of stations sufficiently wide?

Table 3.2 Hypothetical example of how skill areas could be assessed in the 12 OSCE stations

Skill areas	Station 1	2	3	4	5	6	7	8	9	10	11	12
History												
Alcohol dependency	x											
Panic attacks		x										
Assessing risk					x							
Severity of depression									x			
Physical examination												
Fundoscopy				x								
Cranial nerves									x			
Extrapyramidal signs										x		
Mental state examination												
Delusions		x										
Cognitive assessment							x					
Flight of ideas												x
Auditory hallucinations											x	
Communication												
Angry relative	x											
Discussing treatment						x						
Explaining aetiology											x	
Discussion with consultant			x									

27

Table 3.3 Hypothetical example of how content areas could be assessed in the 12 OSCE stations

Content areas	Station											
	1	2	3	4	5	6	7	8	9	10	11	12
Alcohol dependency	x											
Panic disorder					x							
Assessing risk		x										
Depression									x		x	
Raised intracranial pressure				x								
Normal findings								x				
Parkinsonism										x		
Schizophrenia		x	x			x						
Amnestic syndrome							x					
Mania												x

By reviewing the stations in the blueprint this can be ascertained and deficiencies spotted and addressed.

The same principles can be used for a 'station bank'. In this case there would be many more rows of stations in the exemplar Tables 3.2 and 3.3. The examinations panel would use them to establish what areas questions have been written to examine, whether a sufficient breadth and depth had been established and where any deficiencies lay. Another way of looking at the stations would be to consider whether a suitable demographic range had been included (enough stations representing each sex, racial group, socio-economic group and so on).

Structure of the examination

The use of a blueprint also allows the layout of an examination to be properly planned. In the example above, a rest station would need to be added to ensure that no candidates started on station 3 (as the candidates would obviously have to have just completed station 2 before they could attempt station 3). It also ensures that there is not a run of stations assessing one particular skill area (e.g. all the physical examination stations together).

One argument against using OSCEs is that they assess small areas of clinical skills in isolation. The further a student progresses within a medical specialty, the more important it becomes to ensure that he or she is able to integrate skills. This has traditionally been examined in the long case and will continue to be so examined in Part II of the MRCPsych. This sort of assessment is not prevented in the OSCE, as it can be achieved by using 'linked' stations. One example is that of hypothetical stations 2 and 3, above, where two stations were linked to gain insight into a candidate's ability to obtain specific information and then be able to communicate it effectively to a consultant. It would be possible to use more linked stations to assess more complex skills. This to itself increases the complexity of the examination, however, such as the need for 'rest' stations to ensure that candidates always reach the linked stations in the required order.

Validity of the blueprint

A blueprint has been used by other organisations to establish the validity of an OSCE, such as the General Medical Council (GMC) for its Professional and Linguistic Assessment Board (PLAB) examination (Tombleson et al, 2000). The approach used in this instance was to take a bank of questions and send them out to successful examinees and accident and emergency (A&E) specialists. Those contacted were then asked to rate the stations for either frequency seen (examinees) or importance (A&E specialists). This was further validated by examining activity data for A&E attendances and admissions at three hospitals. For this examination the GMC was able to demonstrate that the clinical problems used were appropriate.

That study was retrospective, but it is feasible to look at subject areas prospectively, while adopting some to the approaches used by Tombleson *et al*. Examples would be asking Part I candidates to fill in a diary recording clinical activity, or reviewing trust records of clinical contact (unfortunately these are usually available for admissions only). From this a reasonable idea could be reached of the range of clinical scenarios typically encountered. It would, however, be necessary to establish in addition a list of uncommon clinical conditions that are none the less important owing to their severity.

From such planning studies a schema for an examination can be derived and each of the clinical problems can be examined in a way that taps into the core clinical competencies expected of candidates.

Station development

Once the competencies to be assessed have been defined, the next step is to develop the actual stations. As described, the blueprint and educational objectives must drive this to ensure a balanced and objective examination. Within the process used by the College, the first step is to define the construct. A station's construct sets out its assessment objective. Box 3.2 shows the constructs for stations 2 and 3 in the example described above.

From these constructs those developing the stations can select the appropriate materials. There would be a briefing document for both the role-player and the examiners that sets out the phenomenology and history that the role-player will enact. These scenarios have to cover the information the candidate is expected to elicit, how the role-player should play the part (i.e. how the actor would appear on mental state

---

Box 3.2 Hypothetical constructs for stations 2 and 3

Station 2
The candidate is able to establish the patient's delusions and identify the risk to others arising from them in a concise and focused manner.

Station 3
The candidate is able to communicate succinctly over the telephone to a consultant the findings following examination of a patient, correctly identifying the delusions present and the risk to others arising from them.

---

examination) and also sufficient 'back story' and information to allow the actor to respond to questions in a manner consistent with the role. This must also be sufficient to allow responses to questions that may stray from the intended focus – a not uncommon problem in an OSCE. In the examples above, this scenario would be common to stations 2 and 3, but additional information, including cue questions, would be needed for the examiner in station 3, to allow that person to enact the role of supervising consultant. These briefing documents are vital in ensuring consistency across role-players and thus to ensure that candidates' experience in the examination is standardised. Training and comprehensive description of the role are therefore vital, as highlighted by Tamblyn *et al* (1991).

Reliability over multiple circuits has been demonstrated in clinical examinations (Colliver *et al*, 1991*a*), as has lack of fatigue-induced variability when the actor has to repeat the role many times (Colliver *et al*, 1991*b*). Note that in the College spring 2003 OSCE, role-players played their parts up to 48 times a day and in some cases repeated this over 3 days.

Finally, a mark sheet is drawn up that specifies the domains on which the station will be marked. In the College examination, this usually is limited to four or five domains, each of which is then given a mark on a fixed scale. These scores are used to generate the final mark. The weighting is not known to the examiner. A domain common to the majority of stations is 'Communication'. In stations where assessment of communication skills is part of the construct, it may be given a weighting such that it is the most important domain for that station. For others it may constitute the most minor and in others anywhere in between. The weighting corresponds with the assessment objective defined in the station construct. A final domain of 'Global assessment' is also used. Currently this is used to record the examiner's overall impression of the candidate's performance but it is not used in the final mark. Instead, this rating is used to allow an inference to be drawn as to how accurately the main marking domains and their weightings correspond with the station construct.

Conclusions

The blueprint functions as a starting point in that it allows planning of the collection of stations that make up the bank from which individual examinations are derived. It also is of use as the terminal point in planning both the structure of the examination and the set-up of the stations. Knowledge of how blueprints are used will allow trainers and trainees to generate mock examinations and understand how the overall structure of examinations is arrived at.

References

Colliver, J. A., Robbs, R. S. & Vu, N. V. (1991a) Effects of using two or more standardized patients to simulate the same case on case means and case failure rates. *Academic Medicine*, **66**, 616–618.

Colliver, J. A., Steward, D. A., Markwell, S. J., *et al* (1991b) Effect of repeated simulations by standardised patients on intercase reliability. *Teaching and Learning in Medicine*, **3**, 15–19.

Dauphinee, D. (1994) Determining the content of certification examinations. In *The Certification and Recertification of Doctors: Issues in the Assessment of Clinical Competence* (eds D. I. Newbie, B. C. Jolly & R. E. Wakeford), pp. 92–104. Cambridge: Cambridge University Press.

Royal College of Psychiatrists (2001) *Curriculum for Basic Specialist Training and the MRCPsych Examination*. Council Report, CR95. Gosport: Ashford Colour Press.

Tamblyn, R. M., Klass, D. J., Schnabl, G. K., *et al* (1991) The accuracy of standardized patient presentation. *Medical Education*, **25**, 100–109.

Tombleson, P., Fox, R. A. & Dacre, J. A. (2000) Defining the content for the objective structured clinical examination component of the Professional and Linguistic Assessments Board examination: development of a blueprint. *Medical Education*, **34**, 556–572.

CHAPTER 4

Interviewing skills in the context of the OSCE

Linda Gask and Rosie Illingworth

In the OSCE, the candidate will be given a series of particular tasks to carry out; these could involve any one of taking a specific history, examining a feature of the mental state or providing information about investigations, aetiology, treatment or prognosis. All of these provide opportunities for assessing the quality of doctor–patient communication. The patient may be simulated. In practice this should make no difference to you. Treat the patient as a real patient. Research has shown that simulated patients are rarely distinguished by candidates from real patients anyway (Wallace *et al*, 2002).

Style, content and structure

We can distinguish the *style* of the interview from its *content* and *structure*; a candidate may be assessed on all three of these aspects of communication (see Table 4.1). Specific aspects of content are addressed in the other chapters of this book. In this chapter we provide some key principles to help you to structure the very brief interviewing tasks afforded by OSCE stations, as well as some hints on aspects of style that you may be marked on.

Remember that you will have only 7 minutes at each station. It is important to read the instructions carefully outside each station – you have 1 minute to do so and prepare yourself. Think what the task is asking you to do. Instructions are usually clear and looking for competency in a given domain – for example, 'concentrate on the presenting complaint' means just that. You can be assured that the tasks chosen are relevant and important to your specialty. As Smee (2003) pointed out, the design of an OSCE is usually the result of a compromise between the assessment objectives and logistical constraints. You are unlikely to be faced with an angry, loud patient, as this would be too disruptive for the other stations.

Table 4.1 The three dimensions of an interview

Dimension	Description
Style	Determined by the range and pattern of skills employed by the clinician both in building rapport with the patient early in the interview and in response to what the patient has to say.
Content	What is covered in the interview – this will be partly determined by the range of questions asked by the interviewer but also influenced by what the patient spontaneously offers (or in an OSCE has been primed to ask or offer)
Structure	The overall pattern of questioning and the way in which the interview topics and tasks are organised

The content of the interview is determined not only by the patient but also by the specific topics addressed by the doctor. The quality of the information obtained under each 'topic heading' will be greatly influenced by the skill of the interviewer. So style and structure affect on the final result – what the patient actually says. The skill of interviewing lies in getting the balance right between an 'open-ended', 'checking-out' style of interviewing – which can encourage a patient to talk more, and may be essential in engaging a person who is finding it difficult to express feelings (Hopkinson *et al*, 1981) – and a more 'probing' and systematic style of interviewing – which seems to be important in getting accurate factual information (Cox *et al*, 1981). A skilled interviewer is able to demonstrate flexibility and to switch between styles, as well as to respond to cues provided by the patient. It is also essential to make the discussion appropriate to the patient's cultural context, to avoid jargon and to tailor language to educational level.

Beginning the interview

Before beginning the interview, there are a number of important things to check; these are sometimes termed 'greeting and seating'. You may be marked in an OSCE for carrying out one or more of the following:

- introducing yourself and saying what your role is
- mentioning the patient's name, which both checks the person's identity and gives a positive message of interest
- indicating the purpose of the interview
- explaining how long it is likely to take (about 7 minutes)
- checking that patient is happy about all this.

> **Box 4.1** Quickly establishing the history of a problem
>
> Establish as clearly as possible:
>
> - the nature of the problem
> - the time of onset
> - the development of the problems or symptoms over time
> - precipitating factors or possible links with life events
> - key events since the onset of the problem
> - whether there are alleviating or exacerbating factors, and if so what they are
> - what help has been given or offered
> - what is the *patient's view* of what is wrong and of any help offered so far, and what help the patient would like

If the patient is clearly anxious about seeing a psychiatrist, this should be addressed early, by acknowledging that it might be difficult and saying something like 'How do you feel about talking to me?'

The first couple of minutes of the interview are crucial in demonstrating that you have established rapport (by making eye contact and establishing a conversation) with the patient – which is often specifically looked for by the examiner.

Getting the history of a specific problem: the key tasks

The interviewer should ideally establish as clearly as possible the items in Box 4.1 – but this may be difficult in the time allowed and the task may focus on only one or some of these items.

Eliciting the patient's ideas about aetiology is important because it can help the psychiatrist to understand what may be worrying the patient most. The specific enquiry about symptoms will be determined by the nature of the presenting problem – for example, systematically enquiring about symptoms of major depression, the alcohol dependence syndrome and so on.

Providing information to patients

The main topics about which a candidate may have to provide information include: diagnosis, aetiology, investigations, treatment and prognosis. It is crucial to avoid use of jargon terms and to use words that all patients can understand. Some general guidance is given below.

Diagnosis

The following framework contains the essential skills for discussing diagnosis:

- Establish the patient's perceptions of the problem. What does the patient know already? What are the patient's ideas, concerns and expectations?
- Provide a basic diagnosis. This should be done succinctly.
- Respond to emotions. This is done by making it clear that it is acceptable to talk about feelings and by acknowledging the emotions that are being expressed.
- Provide details of the diagnosis. This involves going on to provide more detailed information, using language that the patient will understand and short sentences that make the point very clearly. Indicate, if you can, whether this is a common problem.
- Check the patient's understanding and elicit questions. Stop frequently to check that the patient understands and ask for questions. Equally, you should also check that you have fully understood the patient's concerns. At the end you should ask the patient 'Do you have any questions about what we have just discussed?'

Aetiology

Once again:

- find out what the patient knows already
- provide information in appropriate language
- check the patient's understanding and elicit questions.

Be prepared to respond to emotional reactions to the information you are providing. Information may be 'bad news' and you must therefore use the skills involved in breaking bad news, particularly giving a 'warning' to alert the patient that things are not straightforward before moving on to provide more detailed information. The patient will usually indicate whether he or she wants to know more, or whether they wish to opt out of deeper discussion at that point.

Investigations

As a general guideline, the interviewer should ensure that he or she explains:

- the purpose of any investigations
- what will actually be done to the patient
- whether the patient should expect any discomfort

- how soon the result will be known
- how the patient will be told the result.

Then ask how the patient feels about the tests. Any fears should be explored and truthful reassurance given. To conclude, the patient should be asked whether there are any further questions; if there are any, these should be answered honestly, without minimising common difficulties.

Treatment

The treatment to be discussed may be a psychological therapy, drug treatment or electroconvulsive therapy (ECT) (see Part II of this book for more information about the specific content of tasks that you must prepare for). The interviewer may be asked to provide the information necessary, for example for a patient to provide consent to treatment.

It is important to check what the patient knows already and indicate a willingness to respond to concerns and to answer questions. Topics to be covered will vary with the nature of the treatment to be given, but patients generally want to know about:

- how treatments work
- how they are actually given (i.e. what the patient will experience)
- how long treatment will go on for
- why the patient is being offered this type of treatment.

Drug treatment

Clear information should be offered and, ideally, each patient should be told for each drug the following information:

- its name
- what it is intended to do
- the dose, route and frequency of administration
- how long the patient should go on taking it (mention should be made of the importance of continuing treatment even after symptoms disappear)
- any special precautions (e.g. to avoid driving or using machinery)
- any interactions with other drugs, foods or alcohol
- possible side-effects and what to do if they occur
- what to do if a dose is missed or extra ones taken
- how to tell whether the treatment is working and what to do if it is not.

This is a lot of information to be given in a consultation and for patients to remember without writing it down. You could offer to supplement a verbal discussion with written information, and to discuss the treatment further with the patient later. Treatment must be explained clearly, without jargon so that, as far as possible, informed consent can be given.

To be sure that there has been no misunderstanding patients can be asked to repeat back what the interviewer has told them about the treatment.

Remember that for women who may be pregnant or intending to become pregnant some drugs must be avoided.

Prognosis

Similar advice applies to providing information about prognosis. The skills here necessitate combining the provision of information that the patient needs to know with, where indicated, the provision of hope and reassurance.

Closing the interview

It is indicative of effective communication skills if you remember to close the interview. Simply saying 'Thank you for talking to me' will suffice as an indicator of the respect between doctor and patient. Remember that, in the OSCE, a bell will ring after 6 minutes at each station. This is to warn you that there is only 1 minute left to complete your task.

Key aspects of interview style

Box 4.2 lists some key aspects of style.

Open-ended questions

These are questions that cannot be answered in one word. A common error in interviewing is to ask too many questions that can be answered only by 'yes' or 'no' too early in the interview, which does not give the patient the opportunity to describe how he or she is feeling. Sometimes

---

Box 4.2 Some key aspects of style

- Asking open-ended questions
- Listening
- Facilitation
- Noticing and responding to verbal cues – clarification
- Noticing and responding to non-verbal cues
- Non-verbal behaviour of the interviewer
- Eliciting and dealing with emotion
- Checking
- Encouraging precision
- Summarising

---

candidates fall back on closed questions because they are worried about having insufficient time. It is actually more effective and time-saving to obtain information through open questions.

Directive questions such as 'Tell me about how you have been sleeping' help to direct the patient to a particular topic without closing down the conversation. Closed questions have their place nearer the end of the interview to fill in gaps in information.

There are some question types to avoid. Multiple questions, especially, are not helpful, such as 'Is there anything that makes it feel better or worse?' This is much more effectively asked as two separate questions and is an example of how a closed question can be used appropriately. Another type of question to avoid is the leading question, such as 'You have been taking your medication, haven't you?' These are unhelpful as you are less likely to get an honest response. There can be a tendency in an examination to move into these types of question when you want to confirm your own thoughts. It is more effective to stick with open questions and receive an answer that comes from the patient.

Listening

Listening is a key skill. It is essential to allow the patient time to talk without interruption, not only at the beginning of the interview but also at crucial points. Silence may be important. However, in the setting of an OSCE the opportunity for demonstrating skills in using silence will be limited because of time pressures! Basically, it is essential to be able to demonstrate enough confidence to give the patient time to reply and not to rush the patient. You will be marked down on aspects of style if you rush the patient or do not give him or her an adequate opportunity to reply. This is where you need to trust the examiners to have set a task that is achievable in the time limit. Hold your nerves in check and focus on the patient. If a moment of silence is appropriate, then pause.

Facilitation

Facilitation refers to encouraging the patient to continue talking, either by verbal means (e.g. saying 'Go on ...') or by non-verbal means (e.g. nodding).

Noticing and responding to verbal cues

Key words and phrases offered by the patient will indicate what he or she is worried about – these are the verbal cues. One way of responding is to ask a question. Another, often more efficient way is to *clarify* what the patient is saying. This may be done by asking, for example, 'What do you mean when you say you have been having panic attacks?' Staying with the patient's own words is often much more efficient than embarking on a checklist of questions about panic attacks immediately.

You may also delay your comment until the patient has finished a particular story, before saying something like 'A moment ago you said you had been depressed before you had this attack. Can you tell me more about that?'

Noticing and responding to non-verbal cues

Such cues include changes in posture or eye contact when talking about particular problems. Commenting on these can be very effective in helping to discover what is worrying the patient, but these comments must be offered with sensitivity (e.g. 'You seemed quite tense when we talked about your father').

Non-verbal behaviour of the interviewer

How well you maintain appropriate eye, contact and posture may also be marked in the OSCE.

Eliciting and dealing with emotion

Making an empathic comment means letting the patient know that you have noticed, or are prepared to offer a suggestion about, what the patient seems to be experiencing. It is important to phrase this as, for example, 'You seem quite upset when you are talking about this' rather than 'You are upset by this'.

When a person is talking about frightening experiences, the flow of conversation may be helped by the use of empathic statements such as 'That must have been very frightening ... you must have wondered what on earth was going on', and this also helps to build rapport and demonstrate empathy.

Checking

Checking allows you to review the information elicited and to correct any misunderstandings. Checking comments also indicates that you have been listening and so helps you to develop rapport. It can also provide useful 'thinking space', during which you can decide what to talk about next.

Encouraging precision

You may need to explain that you need to be as precise as possible about information. Be prepared to say something like 'I'm still not sure that I've got this quite right. Can we try and sort this out before we go any further?' Precision is essential when the task you are carrying out involves taking a history and examining a feature of the patient's mental state. Lack of precision is a common criticism. You will have to decide whether you have you got enough of the right information to be able to come to conclusions about the presence or absence of particular symptoms or a particular psychopathological feature.

Summarising

Summarising statements can be used to check what the patient has reported and to provide a link to the next part of the interview. An example would be 'Can I just summarise what you've told me about the depression? Correct me as I go along.' At the end you could add 'Have I got that right?'

Mental state examination

The candidate needs to be able to clarify the nature of the patient's experience and to get the patient to describe exactly what he or she is preoccupied with or concerned about. This will mean employing precision when, for example, asking about the exact nature of hallucinations and especially when assessing the degree of suicidal risk. Questions should be jargon free and easy to understand but also asked in a sensitive manner. Be absolutely clear how you will question a patient about all aspects of mental state in a sensitive, clear and organised fashion before the examination – this is something that you can easily practise and prepare for in your everyday work. Clarification, obtaining examples of the patient's own words, is also essential when you are asked to establish the quality and severity of mood disturbance and/or to examine the nature and intensity of depressive thoughts.

Therapeutic interviewing skills

It is unlikely that you would be asked to carry out a complicated counselling task at an OSCE station, but you might be asked to, for example, discuss treatment with a patient in order to try to get him or her to stay on medication. There are specific skills involved in trying to help a person to change his or her behaviour – which might include taking medication or stopping something such as smoking or excessive drinking.

Motivation skills

- Be non-judgemental: do not indicate your displeasure at what the patient is choosing to do or not do.

41

- Ask the patient to tell you the advantages and disadvantages, from their point of view, of changing their behaviour.
- Give your opinion in the form of key 'information', as discussed above. Do not simply tell the patient what is best for them. Again, provide opportunities to ask questions.
- Negotiate a plan. Negotiation means reaching an agreement, which might require some give and take on both sides. It is not the same as giving advice.

Structure: the organisation of the interview

Examiners will be concerned not just about the style and content of the interview but also about the general way in which it is structured – is it coherent? Interviewers who move between different topics for no clear reason or who do not appear to be following a clear train of thought will be marked down. It is disconcerting to be on the receiving end of a number of questions without understanding why there has just been a change of topic, for example from depression to appetite. You might keep the patient informed, and therefore more willing to cooperate, by using a *transition statement*, such as 'Now you've mentioned depression, there are a few other important things I just need to ask you about. Can I start off by asking about how your appetite is?' There is a balance, however, to be struck between, for example, asking a systematic list of questions about unusual thought content and being able to pick up cues offered in the interview, which indicates responsiveness to the concerns and worries expressed by the patient.

As you move from station to station, concentrate on the task in hand. You may leave a station and realise you missed an important aspect. There is nothing you can do once the time is up for that station. All the tasks carry equal marks, so it is important to concentrate on earning the points at the next station. The time for review is after the examination has finished. Some candidates even find the OSCE enjoyable!

References

Cox, A., Hopkinson, K. & Rutter, M. (1981) Psychiatric interviewing techniques. Naturalistic study: eliciting factual information. *British Journal of Psychiatry*, **138**, 283–291.

Hopkinson, K., Cox, A. & Rutter, M. (1981) Psychiatric interviewing techniques. Naturalistic study: eliciting feelings. *British Journal of Psychiatry*, **138**, 406–415.

Smee, S. (2003) Skill based assessment: ABC of learning and teaching in medicine. *British Medical Journal*, **326**, 703–706.

Wallace, J., Rao, R. & Haslam, R. (2002) Simulated patients and objective structured clinical examinations: review of their use in medical education. *Advances in Psychiatric Treatment*, **8**, 342–350.

CHAPTER 5

Tips for passing the OSCE

Peter Bowie

The OSCE format exposes the candidate to much greater examiner observation and scrutiny than the previous format of Part I of the MRCPsych examination – the long case and viva, when the examiners observed the candidate with the patient for only 10 minutes. In the OSCE, candidates are observed for much longer (84 minutes) and are required to complete a much more diverse range of tasks. In addition, whether or not a candidate passes depends almost entirely on his or her competence in completing the task. There is minimal, if any, scope for direct interaction between candidate and examiner. This is a simple fact of the OSCE format and there is no point in trying to engage examiners directly unless the station instructions explicitly tell you to do so, as the structured mark sheets allow marks to be awarded only for the task being examined.

Preparation

There are a number of ways that you can prepare for the OSCE.

First, you can prepare a list of potential OSCE scenarios. Remember that any OSCE circuit will be designed to test your ability to take a history, to examine aspects of the mental state, and to give information about a disorder, its treatment and outcome to a patient, a carer or, possibly, a consultant. In addition, you will encounter at least one station requiring a physical examination and there may be stations relating to risk assessment and a patient's capacity to consent to treatment.

There may also be stations where results of investigations are available and you are asked to interpret these and discuss their implications (probably with a patient or carer rather than the examiner). All of these skills could be tested in relation to psychiatric disorders that you are likely to have encountered in your first year of training – in other words, any condition that may present to general or old age psychiatry. Make an exhaustive list.

Box 5.1 Candidate instructions for the cognitive state station

Mr Smith has been referred to you in a psychiatric out-patient clinic because of problems with his memory. Please conduct a cognitive assessment in order to establish the degree of his cognitive impairment.

Having produced a list of potential scenarios, you will need to consider how you would approach each one. Box 5.1 gives an example of a station where you are asked to perform a cognitive state examination – think about what you would want to cover in order to perform an adequate examination of the cognitive state. Note that you are not specifically asked to carry out a mini-mental state examination; instructions would never be this narrow or specific. You would not, for example, be asked to make a rating for a patient on the Hamilton Rating Scale for Depression. You may decide that performing a mini-mental state examination is the best way of tackling this station but beware – does the mini-mental state adequately assess all areas of cognition? It does not assess long-term memory, nor does it assess orientation in person, for example.

Second, you need to practise carrying out the short specific tasks that may be encountered in an OSCE. Obviously, you should practise elements of history-taking and mental state examination, but you should also pay particular attention to explaining the diagnosis, treatment and prognosis of a variety of conditions. You can do this with patients and carers and ask them for feedback. You can ask colleagues, other members of your multidisciplinary team and your consultant to observe you carrying out these tasks. Equally, you could ask team members or colleagues to role-play situations with you while another acts as an observer. An obvious place for short tasks to be observed is the ward round, and another is the clinic if you receive direct supervision with new cases. When practising these tasks you should try to work to time constraints.

Third, you should consider using a video-camera to record short tasks carried out with patients, carers or role-players. You may find it easier working with people role-playing rather than patients, as the former are more likely to keep to the task and time constraint, but not everyone around you will have the ability to act out a role! Having made a video, you then have the opportunity to review this in detail; also review it with your consultant or tutor. Video equipment should be available on all training schemes – if you cannot find it, speak to your College tutor.

Fourth, you should make an effort to observe others interviewing patients and carrying out these short tasks. This often happens in case conferences, ward rounds and in the clinic.

You should start practising these skills sooner rather than later, several months before the examinations. Do not leave it until the period between the multiple-choice written Part I paper and the clinical.

The OSCE by definition involves skills-based assessments, and the circuit of stations is a fair reflection of the basic skills necessary to practise psychiatry, so it would be naive to believe that these skills can be acquired overnight.

When making an exhaustive list of potential stations, you may also consider how these are going to be marked. An example of a mark sheet is available on the College website (see Figure 5.1). You will notice that they all have between three and seven broad items to be marked on a five-point scale (A–E). The final station mark is computed from the marks for each broad item. Usually there will be a mark for communication; it is worth giving some consideration as to what other items are likely to be on mark sheets. This will give you some idea of the range of tasks that you need to cover at a particular station. Failure to carry out a task that is itemised on the mark sheet will mean that you score E for that item; this obviously makes the station more difficult to pass, as you will have to compensate on the remaining items.

The OSCE circuit

The OSCE has 12 stations; there may also be a rest station and one or more pilot stations (i.e. trial ones that don't count towards the score but which have to be attempted by candidates). The stations will be laid out roughly in a circuit, but at some centres there may be some distance between some stations; if you have mobility problems, you should make examination staff aware of this beforehand. Each station stands alone with regard to the final mark and there are no killer stations (see below).

You can therefore afford to do poorly at one station, although this is not recommended! If you do so, you must try to put it behind you. If you pass at the other 11 stations, you will pass the examination. Equally, performing extremely well at one station will not compensate for a poor performance elsewhere, so you should approach each as a mini-examination that has to be passed.

The present format does not include any 'killer' stations (a station that must be passed in order to pass the whole examination). Killer stations are often ones such as cardiopulmonary resuscitation (CPR); even if a CPR station is included in the MRCPsych OSCE, it is unlikely to be a killer station. If killer stations are included in the future, then

EXAMINER MARK SHEET

Station Title: Explanation of schizophrenia to relative

Station Number:

Candidate Number:

Candidate Name:

Examiner Number:

Examiner please mark one lozenge for each objective
Key: A=Excellent, B=good, C=average, D=fail, E=severe fail

CONSTRUCT: The candidate demonstrates the ability to establish rapport with a distressed relative and to explain the aetiology, nature, signs and symptoms of schizophrenia, its treatment on both pharmacological and psychosocial in a way that the relative understands and balances accurate and realistic information with installation of hope.

	A	B	C	D	E
COMMUNICATION	☐	☐	☐	☐	☐
NATURE AND CHARACTERISTIC FEATURES OF SCHIZOPHRENIA	☐	☐	☐	☐	☐
CAUSAL EXPLANATIONS	☐	☐	☐	☐	☐
TREATMENTS AND SIDE-EFFECTS	☐	☐	☐	☐	☐
OUTCOME	☐	☐	☐	☐	☐
ISSUES OF RISK	☐	☐	☐	☐	☐
GLOBAL RATING	☐	☐	☐	☐	☐

Figure 5.1 An example of an OSCE mark sheet. From the College website (www.rcpsych.ac.uk/traindev/exams/regulation/osce.pdf), reproduced with permission.

candidates will be informed in advance. In the absence of such advice, you can safely assume that you can fail at any one of the stations and still pass overall.

During the examination the timing of the stations will be controlled, for example by a bell system or a verbal commentary. You *must* keep to the timing. If you finish a station early, then sit quietly and recap the task that you have just gone through – you may have forgotten to cover something and still have the opportunity to carry it out. If you leave a station early, the examination staff will take you back. This is disruptive and may break your concentration. It is equally important to leave the station promptly at the final signal. If you are in mid-sentence you should simply apologise to the role-player and leave the station – failure to do so will mean that you have less time to read the instructions and gather your thoughts for the next station, and you are unlikely to gain any more marks for spending an extra 15 to 30 seconds in a station.

There will also be a signal to warn you that the station is coming to an end (probably 30–60 seconds before the end). Try to have most of the task completed by this stage and use this time to cover anything else that you consider important.

The role-play

The College has decided not to use real patients in the OSCE; at most stations, therefore, you will be faced with a simulated patient or simulated carer (some stations will feature an interaction between the candidate and examiner only). The role-players performing as patients or carers are professionals and make a living from medical role-play. They are extremely competent, realistic and can consistently play the same scenario time and again. They will have received a detailed script outlining the case that they are to portray; any gaps in their brief are likely to be irrelevancies and they will fill these gaps as they see fit. You should regard the role-players as potential allies. You do not need to tell them that you are sitting an examination and are rushed for time – they already know this. They will not be obstructive unless that is part of the script. If you wish to comment on the limited time available, then you should do so in the context of the station scenario.

For example, there may be a station where the doctor is asked to explain the use of anti-dementia drugs to the daughter of a demented patient; you could start this station by explaining to the daughter that you have only a few minutes because you are needed elsewhere in the hospital, or have to start a clinic. Alternatively, you could just make a general introduction and then get on with the task.

Whenever possible, you should take advantage of the fact that the role-player has had an extensive brief; he or she may have more answers than you do. An example of this is where you are asked to explain a treatment such as ECT to a patient. After introductions you could start this station by asking the patient what he or she already knows about ECT – which, with a bit of luck, may be quite a lot, which makes your task easier, as you will need only to confirm and clarify these points. Of course, the role-player may have been briefed to act as though he or she knows very little, but even so it is worth a try.

The role-player is not the only person acting during the stations. You are required to play the role of the doctor in the given scenario. At some stations this will be easy – as, for example, in the cognitive state examination station in Box 5.1. In this case, after introducing yourself you should say to the patient that they have been referred to the clinic because of memory problems and ask them whether it is alright if you test out their memory.

At other stations it may be more difficult for you to keep to the role but perhaps here it is even more important that you do so. The following station sample instructions in relation to the explanation of schizophrenia to a relative can be found on the College website (www.rcpsych.ac.uk/traindev/exams/regulation/osce2.htm):

'This lady, Mrs Bennett, is the divorced mother of one of your patients, Stephen Bennett, who is a 21-year-old university student recovering from a recurrence (second episode) of a schizophrenic illness. This first presented with an acute onset 3 years ago. He has made a good recovery from both episodes, on both occasions he has been treated with oral haloperidol. He stopped medication one year after the first episode and relapsed 6 months ago. This coincided with his final examinations. He is still registered for his degree with examinations pending. He has had several girlfriends at university, although currently does not have a relationship. Both illnesses were of sudden onset and symptoms included auditory hallucinations and thought withdrawal. His mother is very worried. She has asked to discuss him with you at the outpatient clinic. Her son is willing for you to discuss his case with his mother. Explain the nature of schizophrenia and the long-term prospects for her son.'

To pass this station it is important that you play the part of Stephen Bennett's ward doctor. In normal day-to-day practice you would not discuss the nature and outcome of a patient's illness with a carer unless you had good knowledge of the patient. You must therefore act as though you do. You should not start asking questions to gather more history; in the described situation you would already know it fully. There will be several consequences if you do deviate from the task and start taking more history:

- You will be using valuable time.
- You will not be scoring any marks, as the mark sheet (Figure 1) does not award any marks for history-taking.

- The role-player will have to answer questions that she has not been briefed for; the answers are likely to be irrelevant or, worse, misleading.

General OSCE approaches

You will have 1 minute to read the instructions at each station. Read them carefully and mentally prepare a strategy or task list for the station. You do not need to make notes of the instructions, as they will also be available inside the station; you could, though, make some notes on what you hope to cover in the station.

You need quickly to establish a rapport with the simulated patient or carer. Introduce yourself and address the role-player by name – for example, 'Hello Mrs Bennett, I am Dr —, I work with Dr — and have been involved in your son's day-to-day care.'

Put the patient or carer at ease by explaining the purpose of the consultation using the scenario to get you into the required role – 'You wanted to discuss Stephen's illness with me. Stephen is happy for me to see you. What was it you wanted to know?'

Your aim over the next 6 minutes or so is to have a meaningful exchange with the role player. This means that you have to explain things in lay terms – it is important to avoid jargon. Check that the information that you have given has been understood before you move on to a new point. Do not give too much information at once. It is obviously important to give realistic information, but at the same time you should (in the case cited above) try to instil some hope for the future. If you explain a particular treatment, you should cover side-effects but not list every one from the data sheet – just the common ones.

Take note of the role-player's body language: if he or she is upset or unduly worried by what you are saying, this will be reflected non-verbally, if not verbally. If the role-player indicates more extreme discomfort, then you are in trouble. If this happens, you should apologise and ask what it was that caused the upset. This might reveal a simple misunderstanding that you can quickly clarify. This, of course, takes up valuable time, but failure to react to the person's emotional state will almost certainly result in you failing the station. Furthermore, it is possible that the focus of one or two stations will be how you deal with an angry or very distressed simulated patient or carer. In this case marks will be awarded for how well you diffuse the situation; few or no marks are likely to be linked to other tasks, so in these circumstances dealing with the role-player's distress will score marks rather than detract from other tasks.

Throughout all of this the examiner will have a passive, non-interactive role. Try to put the examiner out of your mind – pretend that he or she is not there (focusing on the role-player will help you do so). If you interview a patient in front of a case conference audience, it is best to focus on the patient and ignore the presence of anyone else. The examiner will assess your ability to carry out the defined task with the role-player – gathering information, eliciting psychopathology and giving information, for example. The examiner cannot award marks for an attempt to show off your knowledge about a subject by covering the minutiae. For example, in the scenario described above, where you are required to explain the diagnosis and prognosis of Mrs Bennett's son, you should keep the explanation simple and centre your efforts on what Mrs Bennett is most concerned about. The inclusion of comments about the season of Stephen Bennett's birth or similar trivia is likely to detract from the core task and could possibly cause Mrs Bennett unnecessary distress, as you are implicitly blaming her for conceiving when she did! Similarly, if you are asked to inform a simulated patient about the side-effects of a treatment, do not include the very rare ones (which are usually nasty) in an attempt to impress the examiner. The reaction of the role-player to being told that a potential side-effect is bone marrow failure is likely to be one of terror, even if you have said it occurs only once in a million cases – you will then need to use up valuable time reassuring the patient and re-establishing some rapport.

The most common statement made by role-players after the pilot OSCE circuits was that the candidates lacked empathy. Having some empathy with the person in front of you will make the interview very much easier. Telling Mrs Bennett that you understand that she 'must be very worried' will help her express those concerns and give you opportunities to explain and clarify aspects of her son's case to her.

Perhaps more important is being able to use empathy in an interview with a patient who has a psychosis. Generally speaking, most psychotic experiences are unpleasant and even terrifying; patients (i.e. role-players) are more likely to elaborate on psychotic experiences if they think that you understand what they are going through. The patient with paranoia who believes that a terrorist organisation is following him is going to be very frightened. If you give him the impression that you think he is mad and you keep firing questions at him that reinforce this perception (e.g. 'Do you ever have the experience that the terrorists are taking the thoughts out of your head?'), he is unlikely to tell you anything; in fact, you might make him more agitated and angry. If, however, you empathise with him by saying that it must be awful that these things are happening, then there is a reasonable chance that he might answer questions such as 'How many of them are there?', 'How do you know they are there?', 'Why are they after you?' and 'Are you being followed (or under surveillance) all the time?' You might eventually reach a point where it is logical to ask if he has ever experienced thought interference.

Approaches to specific OSCE stations

The physical examination

Physical examination stations can roughly be divided into two: those stations with a live participant; and those with a manikin.

The live participant is unlikely to be a patient, for two reasons: first, the examination is usually set up so that two or more identical circuits are running simultaneously and therefore different patients would have to be used across the circuits; and second, it is unlikely that the College would subject real patients to the trauma of repeated examinations. Given, then, that you will be examining a role-player, there are unlikely to be any positive findings. Instead, you will be assessed on your interaction with the simulated patient, the completeness of your examination and the fluidity with which you carry it out. There are a number of simple 'do's and 'don't's.

- Wash your hands first if there is provision to do so. Remember to warm your hands (and stethoscope) before touching the patient.
- Let the patient know that you are going to begin the physical examination. Ask the patient for permission before touching them.
- Do not try to examine the patient through clothing. Ask the patient to remove appropriate articles; only do it for the patient after asking permission (this includes spectacles). *Do not ask the patient to remove underwear* – this will not be necessary.
- Maintain communication with the patient as you go along by explaining what you are doing. For example, if you are carrying out a neurological examination you might say 'I would like to test your muscle strength. Can you squeeze my fingers?'
- If the patient shows discomfort or distress, then show consideration by making an appropriate comment. Do not repeat a distressing procedure unless absolutely necessary.
- Remember to maintain the patient's dignity whenever possible; for example, use drapes where appropriate.

A manikin poses a different problem. The instructions may tell you to speak to the manikin as you would a patient. You may feel silly doing this, but there is likely to be an item on the mark sheet relating to this if it is asked for in the instructions. You will probably be required to tell the examiner what you are finding and to give a running commentary of what you are doing. You are not expected to be a specialist in another field, so, for example, if you have to perform fundoscopy on a manikin, you will need to describe what you can see – perhaps 'exudates at 2 o'clock and haemorrhages at 10 o'clock'. Prepare for this part of the OSCE by familiarising yourself with the instruments, such as the ophthalmoscope. It does not look good if you cannot switch the ophthalmoscope on or cannot get the right beam. If you cannot see anything, try to work out what is wrong – do not be tempted to make it up, as the examiner will be able to see that the light is not on or that it is shining on the cheek rather than the pupil.

CPR stations

CPR stations have been a feature of the GMC PLAB examination (see Chapter 3) and have been used by universities in OSCEs. The GMC found that clinicians as examiners were not reliable for this station and the station was temporarily withdrawn (it has now been reinstated). These difficulties have not stopped the College including a CPR station so far. CPR stations involve a special manikin that can be inflated by the candidate; the examiner takes a reading for the amount of air that is forced into the lungs. it is essential that you are familiar with how the manikin works before you encounter it in the examination room. Find a clinical skills centre that has one and practise on it. At the GMC CPR station, the candidate is expected to enact a real-life resuscitation and to give the examiner a running commentary of what is being done. For an observer, the process is rather amusing to watch, but for everybody else in the examination room it must be extremely disruptive. The station starts with candidates attempting to find a pulse and checking for any respiratory effort; having announced that they have found neither they then state that they are going to call for help. This is followed by the candidates shouting (for realism) 'Help!' several times; they then strike the manikin's chest and start CPR. The station invariably finishes within 4–5 minutes, which gives the candidate time to clear the manikin's airway and relax before the next station.

Paired stations

Paired stations occur where information obtained at one station is carried forward to the next station for a related task. If a circuit includes paired stations, there will be rest stations equal in number to the paired stations. This is because it is impossible for a candidate to start a circuit at the second of a pair of stations. If at the start of a circuit you find yourself at a station with instructions that include references to information obtained at the preceding station, you should alert the examination staff or invigilator immediately.

The instructions at the first of a pair of stations will tell you that the information obtained will be used at the following station. The instructions are likely to advise you to take notes to use at the next station. This is good advice – follow it. Remember, if you perform poorly at the first station, the second station will be very difficult. It is therefore a good idea to familiarise yourself with the types of station that lend themselves to pairing, as there is the potential to fail two stations because of a bad performance on the first.

Any risk assessment station has the potential to be followed by a station where you report your findings to a senior colleague (role-played by the examiner). In these situations the examiner at the second station will have full knowledge of the case at the first, so there is little point in making up findings to fill any gaps that you have left. The examiner at the second station will ask you questions about the case, but he or she will be acting as a senior colleague who is trying to establish a clinical picture and will not be conducting a viva.

Towards the end of the station the examiner may ask you for your opinion as to whether the patient is high, medium or low risk; remember that the mark sheet will not give you any scope to give 'medium high' or 'medium low' as an answer. You will have to be bold and choose one of the three categories, but it is likely to be clear cut and so 'medium' is the least likely to be correct.

Assessment of capacity also has the potential to be a paired station. You could be asked to make an assessment of a patient's capacity to consent to (or refuse) a treatment and then at the following station report your findings to a senior colleague (which could include offering your opinion as to whether or not the patient has the capacity to make the decision).

Conclusions

Wise candidates will start their preparation for the OSCE early. They will practise the basic skills of history-taking, mental state examination, physical examination and information-giving not only as part of their everyday work but by asking others to observe and feedback on their ability. Candidates who develop their skills in this way should have no problem with the OSCE provided that they apply these skills to the tasks set at each station and avoid the pitfalls of trying to impress the examiner rather than communicate with the simulated patient.

CHAPTER 6

Training for the OSCE

Abdul Rahim Patel and Pavan Mallikarjun

In recent times, the assessment of medical education has been revolutionised by the widespread adoption of the OSCE. The OSCE is a timed examination in which students move from one station to the next and demonstrate their ability in various domains, such as history-taking, examination, practical skills and communication skills. At each station, the candidate's performance is rated; the series of stations provides an opportunity for the assessment of the student in many clinical situations, as opposed to the traditional long case, where only one clinical encounter was observed (Hodges, undated).

The use of OSCEs as an examination tool has been extensively researched and found to be of good reliability and validity (Hodges *et al*, 1998). Many of the medical Royal Colleges have introduced an OSCE component into their postgraduate Membership examinations. The Royal College of Psychiatrists has recently introduced an OSCE into Part I of the MRCPsych examination following a comprehensive review and reform of College examinations (Oyebode, 2002). The OSCE will be refined and its validity and reliability improved in the MRCPsych examination as more candidates take it.

The MRCPsych OSCE comprises 12 stations with various scenarios that require the candidate to undertake a particular task. The scenarios are drawn from general adult or old age psychiatry appropriate to 12 months' training in psychiatry. The skills to be tested are history-taking, examination skills, practical skills, emergency management and communication skills.

The aim of the OSCE is to test the clinical and communication skills of candidates and it is designed so that an examiner can observe candidates putting them into practice. These skills are developed during training and the candidate's preparation for the OSCE should not be much different from that for the traditional form of assessment. Owing to the novelty of the OSCE for the three groups of people involved – that is, trainers, trainees and examiners – there need to be guidelines on the training of these groups, to enable appropriate utilisation of the

OSCEs as an assessment tool. The training needs of these groups are distinct and are detailed below.

Training the trainers

Trainers – that is, the educational supervisors of the candidates – need to have a complete understanding of the OSCE in order to be able to assist their trainees in achieving the standards required for success in the examination. Various training methods can be used to contribute towards improving the trainer's knowledge of the OSCE. This training could be provided during the Teaching the Teachers Course for educational supervisors. Some of the methods are described below.

Theoretical background

The OSCE has only recently been introduced into the MRCPsych examination and not many trainers are aware of the reasons behind the increasing use of OSCEs for assessment. Gaining an awareness of the evidence base for the use of OSCEs will be the first step towards the acceptance of OSCEs as an effective means of assessing skills. There are many papers that describe the process of introduction of OSCEs (Hodges et al, 2002; Oyebode, 2002; Wallace et al, 2002). The design of the OSCE stations, as well as their reliability and validity, should be explained clearly to trainers, either by providing literature or by conducting courses. There is some guidance available on creating and improving OSCEs (Hodges et al, 2002; Smee, 2003) and this may also be beneficial to trainers.

A useful guide is available on the Royal College of Psychiatrists' website to educators interested in assessment, wherein all the different assessment processes have been described (www.rcpsych.ac.uk/traindev/uep/assessment/bhodges.htm).

Training using video feedback

Studies have shown that it is possible to teach clinicians how to teach medical students with only brief training (Naji et al, 1986). The videos prepared by the College about the conduct of the OSCE can help trainers to understand the process of the OSCE and can further facilitate training. Vassilas & Ho (2000) have provided a comprehensive review of the use of video feedback for teaching purposes.

Discussion forums

A small group of consultants and tutors can watch a video on the OSCE and then discuss the processes involved. This can further facilitate learning.

Training the trainees

Early in their training, trainees need to be aware of the curriculum on which the examinations are based and the skills that are being specifically tested. The trainees require input from various sources during preparation for the OSCE and training should be a continuous process throughout in their training, rather than just before examination.

Ward-based teaching

As with the teaching for the traditional assessment methods, ward-based teaching for the OSCE will prove very useful to the trainee. The trainers should construct every 'OSCE-able situation' (a term coined by the trainees taking the OSCE to designate a clinical situation that could feature at an OSCE station) into a brief OSCE, observe the trainee undertake that task in the ward, and give feedback. The advantages of such training include the ready availability of patients and the one-to-one feedback. However, it is time-consuming and so requires a great deal of commitment from both the trainers and the trainee. Alternatively, trainers may wish to get the trainee to interview the patient in front of the team and report on this later during the supervision. This approach would have the added value of 'desensitising' the trainee to the interviewing of patients in the presence of colleagues.

Out-patient clinics

Once trainees have seen a new patient in an out-patient clinic, they should present their findings to their trainer. On completion of the presentation, the trainer can give a task to their trainee which should be completed within a specified time. The trainer will watch the trainee complete the given task and give feedback after the consultation is over.

Supervision

The 1-hour weekly supervision period can be used to teach particular skills using an OSCE. Trainers will need to prepare an OSCE scenario beforehand. They can then act as the simulated patient and allow the trainee to carry out the task. Discussion can involve feedback to trainees on their doctor–patient relationship skills. This type of practice has been well received by both trainees and trainers (Brazeau *et al*, 2002) and has improved trainees' ability to take a focused history.

Video feedback

Most psychiatric training rotations have added video feedback sessions to their training programmes (Vassilas & Ho, 2000). This could provide an ideal opportunity to assess clinical and communicating skills and to provide feedback to students. Trainees can be filmed doing an OSCE task and this can be viewed by trainers and other trainees. Feedback can then be given. Providing 'benchmark' videos can improve trainees' self-assessment during practice for OSCEs (Martin *et al*, 1998). The trainers can indentify a set of videos on a single task in which the candididates' performances range in quality from good to poor. Trainees can then use these benchmark videos to assess their own skills on the same task. The trainees will thus be able to evaluate their performance better through this process.

Group practice

Training in small groups is commonly undertaken by students. Peers can act as examiners (Ogden *et al*, 2000) and simulated patients in turn.

Revision courses and mock examinations

A short intensive training course might help students to focus on the skills being tested and provide an insight into their strengths and weaknesses. Mock examinations can help students to identify their anxieties and take steps to overcome them. Revision courses can also be organised with the help of specialist registrars, perhaps based on a 6-station or 12-station mock examination.

MRCPsych academic course

The Part I MRCPsych academic course should be structured to have sessions on OSCE teaching, which should include communication skills. Subject to financial and time constraints, course organisers could conduct mock OSCEs. Apart from the obvious benefit to trainees, this has an educational value for trainers as well, and they should be invited to attend. In Birmingham, 9 hours are dedicated annually to OSCEs. Trainees attending the course are divided into three groups of ten students and each group has a trainer and a specialist registrar simulating the patient. All the trainees perform a 7-minute OSCE station, which is observed by the trainer and the remaining doctors. The trainer then leads a 10-minute feedback session on the task.

Training the examiner

The examiners are central to assessment in the OSCE and the success of the OSCE depends on establishing high levels of interrater reliability. The examiners make a large contribution to the objectivity of the OSCE (Wilkinson *et al*, 2003). The involvement and commitment of examiners is central to the success of OSCEs and can be enhanced by providing appropriate theoretical grounding and video training.

Theoretical background

As with the trainers, the examiners need to be aware of the evidence base for the use of OSCEs. The provision of courses and literature can achieve this objective. The involvement of examiners in station construction has been shown to improve interrater reliability (Wilkinson *et al*, 2003). The examiners should be aware of the skills being assessed and should be given an opportunity to provide input into ways of improving the assessment.

Video training

Videos can be used to provide examiners with knowledge of the conduct of OSCEs. Further, to assess interrater reliability, a set of examiners can be asked to rate the performance of a candidate on video at a particular OSCE station. Group discussions on the assessment of the candidate will improve the reliability of assessments.

Conclusions

The OSCE as a method of assessing a candidate's clinical skills has been introduced into the MRCPsych examination after much consideration, and it appears to be both valid and reliable. The success of the OSCE as an assessment tool will depend on appropriate planning and incorporation of training methods to train the trainers, trainees and examiners. Minor adjustments to the current methods of training the trainers will be of much benefit to their trainees in helping them to prepare for the OSCE. The examiners need comprehensive training to improve the reliability of the OSCE.

Acknowledgements

The authors acknowledge support and advice from Professor Femi Oyebode.

References

Brazeau, C., Boyd, L. & Crosson, J. (2002) Changing an existing OSCE to a teaching tool: the making of a teaching OSCE. *Academic Medicine*, **77**, 932.

Hodges, B. (undated) Assessment of competence of trainees in psychiatry. Available at www.rcpsych.ac.uk/traindev/uep/assessment/bhodges.htm.

Hodges, B., Regehr, G., Hanson, M., *et al* (1998) Validation of an objective structured clinical examination in psychiatry. *Academic Medicine*, **72**, 715–721.

Hodges, B., Hanson, M., McNaughton, N., *et al* (2002) Creating, monitoring and improving a psychiatry OSCE. A guide for faculty. *Academic Psychiatry*, **26**, 134–161.

Martin, D., Regehr, G., Hodges, B., *et al* (1998) Using videotaped benchmarks to improve the self assessment ability of family practice residents. *Academic Medicine*, **73**, 1201–1206.

Naji, S. A., Maquire, G. P., Fairburn, S. A., *et al* (1986) Training clinical teachers to teach interviewing skills to medical students. *Medical Education*, **20**, 140–147.

Ogden, G. R., Green, M. & Ker, J. S. (2000) The use of interprofessional peer examiners in an objective structured clinical examination: can dental students act as examiners? *British Dental Journal*, **189**, 160–164.

Oyebode, F. (2002) Commentary. *Advances in Psychiatric Treatment*, **8**, 348–350.

Smee, S. (2003) ABC of learning and teaching in medicine. Skill based assessment. *British Medical Journal*, **326**, 703–706.

Vassilas, C. & Ho, L. (2000) Video for teaching purposes. *Advances in Psychiatric Treatment*, **6**, 304–311.

Wallace, J., Rao, R. & Haslam, R. (2002) Stimulated patients and objective structured clinical examination: a review of their use. *Advances in Psychiatric Treatment*, **8**, 342–348.

Wilkinson, T. J., Frampton, C. M., Thompson-Fawcett, M., *et al* (2003) Objectivity in objective structured clinical examinations: checklists are no substitute for examiner commitment. *Academic Medicine*, **78**, 219–223.

Part II
Some OSCE scenarios

The chapters in Part II give a series of example stations that might appear in the OSCE. Each scenario starts with the station title. The construct and instructions to the candidate appear within a shaded box. You might wish to spend some time (possibly a minute) thinking about the key tasks after reading the instructions and before proceeding. Then, first, the key points to be covered by the candidate at the station are listed. A suggested approach – which is merely illustrative – to the problem is then set out, with samples of what might ideally be said in four stages of the candidate's exchange with the role-player: the opening, the follow-on, the content (i.e. the part of the interview that addresses the task set in the instructions to candidate) and in closing. Note that these represent only extracts of what would be a full interview, within the 7-minute time constraint.

The following abbreviations are used:

C   candidate
E   examiner, in role-play as a consultant
RP   role-player.

Finally, a few key sources are listed where appropriate, by way of references or further reading for the trainee.

CHAPTER 7

Old age psychiatry

Iain Pryde

Assessment of cognitive state

Construct

The candidate establishes a rapport with the patient, displays appropriate sensitivity, and adequately assesses a broad spectrum of cognitive function – orientation to time and place, registration, concentration, recall, naming, repetition, command, reading, writing and drawing (praxis) – for example using the mini-mental state examination or other appropriate techniques.

Instructions to candidate

Dear Doctor,

Re: Andrew Forest, aged 68
    42 West St, Sydenham, London

Kindly assess the above, whose daughter has contacted the surgery saying she is worried about his failing memory.

Regards,

Dr Smith, General Practitioner

You are the psychiatrist from the local community mental health team for older adults, and are visiting Mr Forest at home in response to the above referral letter. You have reached the stage in your assessment where his cognitive function should be examined.

Please conduct an examination of Mr Forest's cognitive function to estimate the nature and extent, if any, of his cognitive difficulties.

Key points to be covered

- Establish a rapport with the patient and test his cognition in a non-threatening manner, adjusting your approach as necessary if the patient becomes upset. Remember – testing cognition can feel threatening and may reveal deficits which the patient has been trying to hide or ignore.
- Adapt your communication to any difficulties the patient might have, such as hearing, visual or cognitive impairment. Sit so he can see your face as this will help him lip-read; enunciate clearly; use short sentences with few clauses in them (working memory deteriorates with advancing age and cognitive impairment, so the beginning of a long sentence may be lost by the time you reach the end of it).
- Test an appropriately broad range of cognitive functions (as in the construct). It may be easier to use a standardised instrument such as Folstein's Mini Mental State Examination (MMSE) – learn this off by heart, and remember that there is a standardised method of administering and scoring it.
- If not using a standardised instrument, be sure that you test a broad enough range of functions with questions of your own.
- Focus on what the question is asking. For example, the MMSE is appropriate here as you are being asked broadly to test cognitive function, but if the history had suggested frontal impairment, which the MMSE does not test, you would have to have memorised a specific frontal test. If you had been asked only to 'test his memory', then you would need to have broadened the range and depth of the memory questions and not be diverted in assessing orientation, praxis and so on.

Suggested approach

Opening

C: So, we've been talking a bit about your memory. Normally when I'm seeing someone who might be having memory trouble, I have a list of questions I ask to see how their memory is doing. It takes about 5 or 10 minutes. Would it be OK for me to ask you these questions just now?

RP: Well, I don't know – how difficult are they?

C: Some are easier than others; some might even seem a bit silly, but I ask everyone the same ones. Just have a go, and if a question's too difficult, don't worry – it's not a test.

RP: OK, fair enough.

Follow-on

C: Thank you. Can I start by asking you what day it is today?

Content

Remember if using the MMSE that there is a standard way of asking the questions. You may not help the patient with the answers, but you should encourage the patient to attempt the questions and remain positive and non-threatening even if he or she get things wrong. For example:

C: A few moments ago I gave you a list of three objects to remember. Can you tell me what they were?

RP: No, no, they've gone.

C: Have a go. Can you remember one of them?

RP: I don't know. ... Was it a ball?

C: Absolutely! Well done. Can you remember any of the others?

RP: Flower?

C: No, flower wasn't one of them. Any other guesses?

RP: [*Pause*] No, no, they've absolutely gone. I just can't remember them. That's terrible – I feel so stupid!

C: Don't worry about it – lots of people have that problem. You got one right, which is great. The other two were 'flag' and 'tree'. Let's just try the next question.

Closing

There may be time for the patient to ask how well he or she did. Answer honestly but tactfully and positively.

C: That was the last question, so we've finished now. Thank you very much for doing that for me.

RP: How did I score? I don't think I did too well.

C: That's OK. I know some of the questions were a bit difficult for you. A lot of people find the same. There were one or two problems with you remembering things, like the three words that I gave you. I think you noticed that at the time. But you did very well on other parts, like giving me your address and drawing those shapes at the end. So no need to feel bad about it!

Sources

Folstein, M. F., Folstein, S. E. & McHugh, P. R. (1975) 'Mini-mental state'. A practical method for grading the cognitive state of patients for the clinician. *Journal of Psychiatric Research*, **12**, 189–198.

Lishman, W. A. (1997) *Organic Psychiatry* (3rd edn). Oxford: Blackwell Science. (For detailed descriptions of cognitive assessment.)

Molloy, D. W., Alemayehu, E. & Roberts, R. (1991) Reliability of a standardized mini-mental state examination compared with the traditional mini-mental state examination. *American Journal of Psychiatry*, **148**, 102.

Collateral history in a case of dementia

Construct

The candidate obtains a collateral history from the relative, covering onset, duration, course, nature and extent of symptoms and their functional sequelae.

Instructions to candidate

Mrs Tomkins is a single lady in her 80s currently on a medical ward, who was admitted 3 weeks ago with a chest infection. She has no other medical problems. The medical staff are concerned that she appears to have memory difficulties, which have persisted in spite of her full recovery from her acute illness. They have asked you, as an old age psychiatrist, for your opinion on her diagnosis.

Mrs Tomkins has denied all symptoms when speaking with you, is bright in mood and though she scored 12 out of 30 on the MMSE she denied any memory difficulties and said she was doing fine at home.

Her niece, Mrs Barbara Morgan, happens to be visiting her aunt and has agreed to speak to you. Mrs Tomkins is happy for you to do so.

Please use the opportunity to obtain a collateral history of Mrs Tomkins' cognitive difficulties to help you with your diagnosis.

Key points to be covered

- Introduce yourself and explain your involvement and why you have asked to speak to Mrs Morgan; thank her for her time.
- Sensitively establish the nature of their relationship and amount of contact, so you may judge how to weight her account.
- Establish whether she or anyone else in the family has noticed memory or similar problems in her aunt. Remember to try to go from open to closed questioning, and summarise and recap to check you are getting it right.
- If the onset is difficult to date precisely, ask when she was last her old self. Cognitive difficulties may come to light following a discrete event but be evident in retrospect for some time before this.
- Offer probes for evidence of cognitive problems if necessary, such as getting lost, losing things, not recognising people, missing appointments, day/night disorientation, loss of skills (e.g. cooking) or difficulty finding words.

- Enquire about the onset (was it obvious and sudden or gradual and insidious, and were there any triggers?), duration, course (fluctuating, progressive, stepwise, stable?) and extent of symptoms. Are there diurnal variations or other things that make it better or worse?
- Remember to enquire about the non-cognitive symptoms of dementia, such as personality change, poor judgement, apathy, irritability, affective features, behavioural disturbance, delusions and hallucinations.
- Crucially, try to assess the functional implications of symptoms – how are they affecting how she is managing at home?
- Have there been any risky behaviours, such as getting lost at night, leaving the gas on, letting strangers into the house?
- Screen for affective disorder, substance misuse and a psychiatric history.

Suggested approach

Opening

C: Thanks very much for seeing me, Mrs Morgan. I'm Dr —. I'm a psychiatrist from the local older adults mental health team, and your aunt's doctors here on the ward have asked me to see her because they think she's having some memory problems.

RP: I see, yes.

C: Now, your aunt doesn't feel she's having any difficulty, but I thought I'd ask whether you might have a different point of view, perhaps?

RP: Oh, certainly. I know she'd say she's fine, but her memory's just not what it used to be.

Follow-on

C: That's very helpful to know. Tell me, do you see much of your aunt normally?

RP: Oh yes, we're a big Jamaican family, lots of aunts and nephews and nieces, so we're always popping in and out. My aunt's almost like a mother to me, really. I see her most days.

Content

C: And you've seen some changes in her, you say?

RP: Oh yes. She's changed quite a lot.

C: When was she last her old self?

RP: Well, she got a lot worse after my mum died a couple of years ago, because they were very close, but to be honest she's been going slowly down hill for the past 4 or 5 years.

C: I see, so quite some time then. And what sort of changes have you noticed?

RP: Well, looking back, I suppose the biggest sign was that she stopped doing as much organising as she used to do. She was always cooking big meals and everything for the family, and we noticed she wasn't doing that any more.

C: So that was quite unusual?

RP: Yes. At first we thought she was just a bit, you know, slowing down, getting old and what have you, but when we tried to encourage her we found she just couldn't do it as well. She got things muddled up and it really frustrated her.

Closing

C: So, can I just check I've got this right? It sounds like she was a very active, sociable person but things have been getting slowly worse for her over the past 4 or 5 years, with a bit of a jump when your mum died but otherwise just slowly but steadily?

RP: That's right, yes.

C: And you say now her memory's poor, she loses things, she can't do stuff like she used to?

RP: Like cooking and cleaning, yes.

C: And you have to prompt her with getting dressed and remembering to eat and so on?

RP: Yes, but, like I say, there's plenty of people around to help out, and she's not doing anything to put herself at harm or anything, so we've been quite happy just supporting her within the family. Do you mind if I go and see her now? She'll be wondering where I am.

C: Not at all – you've been very helpful. I've a much better idea of what's going on now. Thanks very much for your time, and we'll hopefully speak again later.

Explaining dementia to a relative

Construct

The candidate establishes a rapport with the relative and discusses the diagnosis in an honest and realistic but sensitive manner, showing good communication skills and judgement in use of language. The candidate should allow appropriate opportunity for the relative to ask questions, and should deal empathically with any emotional reaction to the news.

Instructions to candidate

You are an old age psychiatrist seeing Mrs Winters in the out-patient department. Her husband, John, is 76 and has recently been diagnosed with vascular dementia. He has an 18-month history of stepwise cognitive decline on the background of hypertension, diabetes and transient ischaemic attacks. His memory is poor, he is apathetic and he needs supervision and prompting with his daily activities, which his wife now does for him. His computerised tomography (CT) brain scan showed extensive small-vessel disease and one or two small infarcts.

Mrs Winters has asked to see you in clinic as she is aware that her husband's memory has been poor and that he has had some tests, but she does not yet know the diagnosis.

Please discuss with Mrs Winters her husband's diagnosis of vascular dementia.

Key points to be covered

- Introduce and set the scene.
- Find out what Mrs Winters understands about her husband's condition – does she have an opinion on what is wrong?
- Pitch your language appropriately, so you do not patronise on the one hand or overwhelm with jargon on the other.
- If necessary, build up to the diagnosis by summarising the problems with his memory and so on.
- Introduce the diagnosis of dementia and allow her to respond. Ask what she understands by the term.
- Sympathetically address any important errors in her understanding, and if appropriate explain what dementia means, and relate this to her husband.

- If appropriate, explain about the type of dementia – but avoid overloading Mrs Winters with information.
- Deal empathically with any emotional reaction to the diagnosis.
- Ask if she has any questions or worries you can help with.
- Explain briefly what happens now – follow-up and so on.
- Allow for future questions.

Suggested approach

Opening

C: Good afternoon Mrs Winters, my name is Dr —. I understand you would like to talk today about your husband John, is that right?

RP: Yes, doctor. I want to find out once and for all what exactly is wrong with him.

Follow-on

C: Of course – you must have a lot of questions. I'll try my best to help answer those today. Tell me, have you had any thoughts yourself about what might be the matter?

RP: Well, at first I thought it was just old age, getting forgetful, you know. But after he had those mini-strokes it got a lot worse and I started to worry if something was, you know, wrong in the head.

Content

C: Yes, his memory's quite a lot poorer, isn't it? Well, you're right in thinking that this is more than just normal ageing, because there have been other changes too, haven't there?

RP: Yes. He's not the same person he used to be. What is the matter with him, doctor?

C: Well, you know we've been talking to you and him a lot, and we've also done a number of tests. Putting all this together, we think he has a condition called vascular dementia. Have you heard of dementia before, or perhaps known of anyone who has that condition?

RP: Well, they said my aunt had Alzheimer's – is that what you're talking about?

C: In a way – Alzheimer's is a sort of dementia, though a different sort from what your husband has. What does dementia mean to you?

Closing

C: I'm afraid we're going to have to stop soon, and I know this has been a lot to take in. Is there anything else you'd like to ask just now, or anything I can help with?

RP: I don't think so, but to be honest I don't think I'm thinking too straight.

C: Of course, it's difficult news to hear, isn't it? Well, I would quite understand if you didn't remember all we talked about today, or if more questions occurred to you after we've finished, so perhaps you'd like to come to see me again next week and I'd be more than happy to talk further. And of course, you can talk to John's keyworker any weekday just by calling the team.

Medication and management in Alzheimer's disease

Construct

The candidate discusses in a positive but realistic manner the management options available, covering both biological and social interventions, and shows good communication skills and use of language.

Instructions to candidate

You are an old age psychiatrist on a home visit to see Mr Robin Page, whose father, Albert Page, is 80, lives with him and has been diagnosed by your consultant as having Alzheimer's disease. Albert has a 3-year history of insidious cognitive decline, with forgetfulness, difficulty finding words, irritability and a deterioration in personal skills, such that the son is having to take on more day-to-day running of the house.

The diagnosis has been discussed with both men. Albert is unable to recognise that he is having difficulties, but has said he is happy for things to be discussed with his son. When last tested, he scored 19 out of 30 on the MMSE. He has no other known medical problems.

Your consultant has asked you to visit Robin Page to discuss what treatment options are available. Albert is not at home, having gone out to place a bet nearby.

Please discuss with Robin the management options available.

Key points to be covered

- Introduce and set the scene – remember that this visit is supposed to be taking place at home, so ask for permission to sit, and so on.
- Remember that sensitive communication and appropriately pitched, non-jargon language should be used.
- Be honest and realistic but sensitive and allow room for hope and a positive attitude.

- Find out whether Mr Page has questions, or any misconceptions that need clearing up.
- Discuss biological and social interventions, aimed at both his father and himself.
- Biological interventions might include acetylcholinesterase inhibitors and symptomatic treatments of other neuropsychiatric complications, such as agitation or psychosis (with, for example, sedatives or antipsychotics).
- Currently in the UK, prescription of acetylcholinesterase inhibitors (donepezil, galantamine, rivastigmine) is done under guidelines issued by the National Institute for Clinical Excellence. It is important to know about these guidelines or if they have changed, what (if anything) has replaced them.
- Social interventions may be multidisciplinary and inter-agency: keyworker support for Albert and his son; help with personal care, housework, shopping; meals on wheels; home adaptations; clubs, day centres, respite; advice on benefits and so on.
- An assessment by an occupational therapist or social worker may be useful.
- You should mention the availability of non-statutory agencies such as a local carers' network for the son or the Alzheimer's Society. Do not overload Mr Page with offers of help or potential sources of it, however, or you will just cause confusion – know what is available, and tailor advice to the individual circumstances.
- Ultimately, stress the need to compensate for any impairments Albert may have now or in the future, while maximising his independence and autonomy in those areas where he remains competent, either independently or with support.

Suggested approach

Opening

C: Good morning, Mr Page. I'm Dr —. Is it OK if I sit here?

RP: Of course, doctor, go ahead.

C: Thank you. Now, my consultant has asked me to come and discuss your father's care with you – is that what you'd like to talk about?

RP: Yes. We've been told he has Alzheimer's disease, but I'm not sure what can be done about it. I've heard there are new treatments available to make it better. Is that right?

Follow-on

C: There are certainly new tablets around which can help some people, but I'm afraid they're not the wonder drugs they might seem from some of the publicity. What have you heard about them yourself?

RP: Oh, just stuff from the papers, 'New cure for Alzheimer's', that sort of thing. Are you going to tell me they aren't any good?

C: No, I wouldn't say that. There are certainly people who benefit from these new tablets. But not everyone does, and even in those who do, their benefits can be quite limited and have to be kept in perspective. I'm afraid it would certainly be wrong to suggest we have anything that can 'cure' Alzheimer's disease. But there is certainly a lot we can do to maximise your father's quality of life, and to help you in caring for him. Tablets may have a role to play in that or they may not, but why don't we start by discussing what's out there?

Content

C: I guess since you've mentioned these new tablets we should perhaps discuss them first?

RP: Yes – I'm still keen to find out about them. What do they actually do if they don't cure the disease?

C: The idea with these tablets is that they change the level of a certain chemical in the brain that's thought to be low in Alzheimer's disease. You may be aware that people's memory and so on usually gets steadily worse in Alzheimer's – have you noticed that in your father?

RP: Yes, that's certainly true – he just gets slowly worse as the months go by.

C: Well, in people who respond to these tablets – and so far we can't really predict who will respond and who won't – they appear to be able to delay the worsening of symptoms for a bit – perhaps a number months or longer.

RP: When you say delay, do you just mean it's putting things off, and they'll eventually start to get worse again?

C: Yes. As far as we know, these tablets don't seem to be able to alter the course of the illness, as such, so people do usually start getting worse again at some point, even if the tablets worked for them in the first place. But it can still be a useful benefit, keeping them more independent for longer than they would have been otherwise.

Closing

C: We're unfortunately running out of time for just now. Are there any other questions I can help with before we sum up?

RP: No. I'll need to mull things over a bit first I think.

C: Of course – you can always ask next time. So, just to recap, we've discussed the new tablets on the market, as well as the older tablets that we sometimes use to help with certain individual symptoms, such as antipsychotics and so on. But just as importantly, we've talked about the very practical things that can help your father keep his independence for as long as possible and help make caring for him easier for you.

RP: Yes. I guess I was quite focused on the idea of this new treatment, but it's nice to know there's other help available as well.

Source

National Institute for Clinival Excellence (2001) *Guidance on the Use of Donepezil, Rivastigmine and Galantamine for the Treatment of Alzheimer's Disease*. Available at www.nice.org.uk/Docref.asp?d=14412.

Variations

Four possible scenarios from old age psychiatry have been described, all involving dementia. Only one of them involves talking directly to the patient, but you might equally reasonably be asked to explain the diagnosis or treatment options to the person with dementia himself or herself rather than a relative.

Other possible scenarios in old age psychiatry include frontal lobe signs on examination, explaining to a relative specifically about Alzheimer's disease, taking a history in the context of depression and physical problems, assessing capacity to consent, and testamentary capacity in the context of dementia. Remember that dementia does occur in people under the age of 65; equally, older people also suffer from depression, psychosis, anxiety disorders and substance misuse (particularly alcohol misuse). In general, bear in mind the greater likelihood of complicating physical illness, drug interactions and sensory as well as cognitive impairment (dementia or delirium) and think of the particular sorts of losses that tend to cluster in old age (bereavement, loss of physical independence, etc.). Finally, do not forget the importance of functional assessment (activities of daily living) and social support – and watch out for implicit ageism, which will get you marked down!

CHAPTER 8

Substance misuse

Hugh Williams

Alcohol history

Construct

The candidate should obtain a brief history of the patient's current drinking and establish whether the patient is dependent, the nature and severity of any physical withdrawal and current alcohol-related problems. A sensitive, non-judgemental interview style should be adopted.

Instructions to candidate

Mrs Jones is a 55-year-old married woman who has been referred to the out-patient department by her general practitioner (GP). Mrs Jones admits that she feels that she may have a serious drink problem and is eager to discuss her drinking and seek help.

Please obtain a brief alcohol history from this patient.

Key points to be covered

- You should be empathic and non-judgemental.
- Introduce yourself to the patient and explain that you wish to obtain a brief history of the patient's recent drinking.
- Encourage the patient to describe her usual drinking pattern (e.g. a typical drinking day, or whether it is episodic binge drinking).
- Establish the number and type of drinks per day or week (in units of alcohol).
- Check for features of alcohol dependence syndrome (according to ICD-10 or DSM-IV criteria).

- Ask about the nature and extent of symptoms of physical withdrawal (e.g. tremors, sweats, hallucinations, seizures, delirium tremens).
- Establish whether there are any alcohol-related problems in terms of physical health, mental health (include suicidal thoughts) or social and family life, and any occupational, financial or legal problems.
- Give feedback to the patient.

Suggested approach

Opening

A clear, empathic, non-judgemental style should be adopted, as often patients may feel ashamed about their drinking. In this case you are aware in advance that the patient has clear concerns and so a simple opening question may suffice.

C: Good afternoon, Mrs Jones. My name is Dr —. Your GP has referred you along here today and I gather there are some concerns about drinking.

RP: Yes, that's right doctor.

C: How do you see things?

RP: I am worried that I might be drinking too much. I find it hard to cut down and just can't seem to stop. Do you think I'm an alcoholic?

Content

Try to establish the number of units of alcohol consumed in an average week and the type of drinking pattern.

C: I would like to hear a little bit more about your drinking. Why don't we begin by you telling me about a recent typical drinking day?

RP: I drink in the morning and throughout the day. It is usually wine but sometimes vodka.

C: So how much might you drink over the course of the whole day?

RP: Perhaps three or four bottles of wine and a few vodkas. Usually a bottle of vodka will last me the whole week.

C: So how many days in the last month would you have had a drink?

RP: If I am going to be honest, doctor, I'm afraid it's been most days for years.

Aim to establish whether dependence criteria are met. If the patient does not volunteer these spontaneously, they should be specifically enquired about. The patient should be asked particularly about the nature and severity of physical withdrawal symptoms. For instance, you will already have established that the patient consumes a very large amount of alcohol (tolerance), is drinking daily (compulsion, stereotypical pattern) and that she finds it difficult to stop or cut down (loss of control). Other evidence of alcohol dependence syndrome and the nature and severity of withdrawal phenomena might be enquired about.

C: You mentioned that you start drinking in the morning. How do you normally feel before you have your first drink?

RP: Oh, I am in bad shape usually.

C: In what way? Do you have any unpleasant physical experiences?

RP: Oh yes. I am normally very jumpy and anxious and my hands shake a lot. Often it is not too bad after I have had my first drink. Sometimes I can't face eating anything and often want to vomit but nothing seems to come up. Maybe it is the weather or the central heating but I tend to perspire a lot. Sometimes my nightdress is soaked.

C: Other patients have told me that sometimes they see things, like insects or animals that aren't really there. Has anything like that ever happened to you?

RP: Oh no – I've never had anything like that!

To assess the nature of any other alcohol-related problems you might ask an open-question like 'Do you feel your drinking is causing any other problems for you?' This might be followed by more direct questions, such as 'How do your family view things?' or 'Do you feel your family life has suffered because of your drinking?'

RP: I don't seem to want to do anything but drink these days. I used to have hobbies and interests. My poor husband is at his wit's end; it is really affecting him too. We don't go out anymore. Although he hasn't said it, I think he might be thinking of leaving me.

Closing

Summarise and feedback.

C: Thus far you have told me that you are worried about your drinking and ...

Offer thanks, affirmation and support to the patient.

C: Thank you for coming along today and being so frank with me. I realise that it must have been very difficult for you. Well done.

A more comprehensive drinking history (e.g. the patient's chronological pattern drinking over years, possible precipitants of drinking, previous treatment) is not expected of the candidate in the time allowed.

Sources

Ashworth, M. & Gerada, C. (1998) Addiction and dependence. In *The ABC of Mental Health* (eds T. Davis & T. K. J. Craig), pp. 43–45. London: BMA Books.

Goldberg, D. (ed.) (1997) Alcohol and drinking problems. In *Maudsley Handbook of Practical Psychiatry* (3rd edn), pp. 194–197. Oxford: Oxford Medical Publications.

Miller, W. & Rollnick, S. (1991) *Motivational Interviewing: Preparing People to Change Addictive Behaviour.* New York: Guilford Press.

Explaining alcohol detoxification to a relative

Construct

The candidate should demonstrate an ability to communicate the fundamental elements and rationale of the alcohol detoxification process to a concerned relative in a confident, caring and understandable (non-technical) manner.

Instructions to candidate

Mr Brown is a 58-year-old unemployed labourer with a long history of severe alcohol dependence syndrome. He has been admitted acutely for in-patient alcohol detoxification. Before admission, he had been consuming in excess of one bottle of spirits per day. In the past, during periods of untreated alcohol withdrawal, he has experienced confusion, fits and delirium tremens.

You are the psychiatric senior house officer on duty and Ms Brown, the patient's 30-year-old daughter, has asked to speak to you regarding her father's treatment.

Please explain the process of alcohol detoxification to this relative.

Key points to be covered

- Engage in clear, empathic communication with this relative.
- The nature of alcohol withdrawal should be explained, including its major complications (e.g. seizures, delirium tremens, Wernicke's encephalopathy).
- Explain the aims of detoxification.
- You should include the rationale of prescribing sedative medication (e.g. benzodiazepines) and the reasons for the use of high-potency B vitamins parentally.
- State the nature of additional measures (e.g. monitoring and treatment of concurrent conditions) and approximate length of the process (e.g. 7–10 days).

- Explain briefly what happens after detoxification (e.g. maintenance of abstinence).
- Respond appropriately to any further concerns or enquiries.

Suggested approach

Opening

You should enquire with an open-ended question what concerns Ms Brown has and try to establish her level of understanding.

C: Good morning Ms Brown. My name is Doctor —. I understand that your father has just been admitted to Rose Ward.

RP: Yes doctor. I am glad he is finally having something done about his drinking.

Follow-on

C: I gathered you would like to talk about your father's treatment and I am happy to try to explain things to you. Have you any particular concerns?

RP: They say that he is going to have a detox but I am not too sure what that means.

Content

You should explain the nature of severe (untreated) alcohol withdrawal and discuss the rationale of the assisted (medicated) withdrawal. The relative should be assured that the patient will receive adequate doses of a sedative (e.g. benzodiazepines), which will then be gradually tapered to zero. The rationale for patients receiving a high dose of the B vitamin complex (e.g. thiamine) by injection should also be explained.

C: Detoxification, or detox for short, is the first step in your father's treatment. It aims to help him stop drinking and reduce any unpleasant withdrawal symptoms or medical complications that sometimes happen in people who have been drinking very heavily.

RP: When he tried to stop drinking in the past he became very confused and started to see things like rats in his bed. Will that happen this time?

C: What you are describing are what we call delirium tremens or DTs, which can sometimes make it difficult for heavy drinkers to stop drinking without medical help. We will be giving your father some medicines to try to prevent these unpleasant things happening to him.

RP: What type of medicines?

C: We will give him some sedative (or Valium-type) drugs for a few days to keep him comfortable and then we will tail off the tablets over the next week or so. We will also be giving him some vitamin injections.

RP: Vitamins? Is that because you think he has not being eating so well recently?

C: Yes and also to try to prevent memory problems that can sometimes happen in heavy drinkers.

RP: I see. What else will his treatment involve?

C: He will be monitored very closely, especially for the first few days, by the nursing staff. He will be encouraged to drink plenty of fluids and take things easy for a few days. We will treat any medical problems that might develop, for instance if he got an infection or something like that.

RP: I see. Does that mean, then, that he won't ever drink again?

It should be explained that detoxification is the first step in initiating abstinence from alcohol but that ongoing treatment will be needed in order to maintain abstinence.

C: As I said earlier, detoxification is just the first part of your father's treatment. It's about, if you like, helping him get off alcohol. The next part will be aimed at helping him maintain his abstinence or stay off alcohol. This involves different types of treatment, such as individual talk therapy or group therapy or attending self-help groups like AA. However, we will talk to him about that later on in the week, when he is feeling a bit better in himself.

Closing

You should allow time to respond to any further concerns by the relative.

C: Is there anything else you would like to ask me or that you are not sure about?

RP: You said you would be giving him Valium-type medicines and I've heard these can be habit-forming. Will he get addicted to them?

C: Yes, you are quite right, these types of drugs can be addictive, but I don't think that will happen in your father's case. He will only be getting them for a short time and they will be gradually tailed off and stopped.

RP: Thank you doctor. I am a bit clearer on things now.

C: Good. You've had a lot to take in. If any other questions come to mind or you want things explained further, you can always contact me or one of the team here at the hospital.

Sources

Chick, J. (1996) Medication in the treatment of alcohol dependence. *Advances in Psychiatric Treatment*, **2**, 249–257.

Kosten, T. R. & O'Connor, P G. (2003) Management of drug and alcohol withdrawal. *New England Journal of Medicine*, **348**, 1786–1794.

Assessing a heroin user – taking a brief drug history

Construct

The candidate should demonstrate the ability to take a brief drug history of the patient's current opiate use in a non-critical, non-judgemental, empathic manner. The candidate should establish the nature and extent of recent drug use, whether physical dependence is present and the nature of any of drug-related problems. As heroin users commonly use or are dependent on other, non-opiate substances, some attempt to establish concurrent drug use (e.g. of benzodiazepines, stimulants, alcohol) should be made.

Instructions to candidate

Mr Smith is a 27-year-old single man who works as a chef. He is currently in the A&E department awaiting transfer to a medical ward for the treatment (incision and drainage) of a large abscess on his left arm. He has disclosed to A&E staff that he is a heroin user and fears that he will experience opiate withdrawal (abstinence syndrome) if he does not receive opiate medication.

You are the senior house officer on duty and have been asked by A&E staff to review the patient.

Please take a brief substance use (drug) history from this person.

Key points to be covered

- Adopt a concerned, empathic, non-judgemental approach to the patient
- Establish the amount, frequency, route of administration and pattern of use of heroin (and other opiate drugs) in the preceding 4 weeks, and elicit features of the opiate dependence syndrome.
- Ask about drug-related problems, including overdoses, as well as about the use of other classes of (non-opiate) drugs.
- Give feedback to the patient and respond appropriately to any further concerns or enquiries.

Suggested approach

Opening

'Heroin addicts' are often depicted as challenging and manipulative individuals who make excessive demands on care staff. Nevertheless, a non-critical, non-judgemental, empathic interview style should be adopted. This will enhance meaningful intercourse and aid in the assessment process.

C: Hello Mr Smith. My name is Dr —. I've been asked by colleagues to come and talk to you about your heroin use.

RP: Listen doc, I've had no gear today and I'm starting to cluck [experience opiate withdrawal] badly. When am I going to get something?

Follow-on

C: I understand that you may be distressed and uncomfortable right now, but before I can decide things I need to find out a little more about your drug use. Would that be alright? It won't take long.

RP: OK doc, but make it snappy – I'm not a happy bunny right now.

Content

Start by asking about drug use in the preceding 30 days. This should include not only heroin but also other opiate preparations. Establish the average daily doses, routes of administration and pattern of drug use (e.g. whether daily or less frequent), as well as whether physical dependence is present.

C: I'd like you to tell me first about your recent heroin use, say over the past 30 days. How often do you use heroin and how much do you usually use?

RP: I've been using heroin on and off for years. I started using again 10 months ago. Right now I'm using up to a gram every day.

C: What way do you use your heroin?

RP: How do you think? I'm injecting – that's why I've got this fucking abscess.

C: Has there been any time in the past month when you've not had heroin? Do you get withdrawal?

RP: You're so right I do. It's like the way I am feeling now. Sweaty, shivery, sick, aches and pains everywhere, feeling really crap and I get the shits [diarrhoea]! I usually take some DF118 [dihydro-codeine] if I can't get heroin and that holds me.

As many opiate misusers use other classes of drugs (e.g. benzo-diazepines, alcohol, cocaine) you should make some brief enquiry in this regard.

C: I'm clear about your heroin use. Can I ask you now if you use any other types of drugs, like benzos, or cocaine or alcohol?

RP: I take crack once or twice a month. I don't take anything else and I don't drink. My father was an alcoholic.

Possible complications of the patient's drug use should be asked about. It may be helpful specifically to cover the following areas of the patient's life: physical health, mental health, social/family life, occupational/financial and legal matters. It is particularly important to enquire about recent overdoses.

C: So far you've told me that injecting heroin has caused this abscess, which needs treatment. Is your drug use causing any other problems for you?

RP: It's costing me £40 a day, every day! I'm having to pop out from work to buy it and the boss is beginning to get suspicious.

C: Have you ever gone over [overdosed] on heroin?

RP: Seen it happen to lots of friends but it's never happened to me.

Closing

Time permitting, a brief summary of your assessment should be fed back to the patient for clarification and the patient thanked.

C: Well, thank you for talking to me. What you've told me so far is ... I'll just need to check the results of your urine test and then I'll talk to the other doctors about your treatment. I've asked you a lot of questions; have you any questions for me?

RP: They are not going to leave me in pain are they? They know I'm a heroin addict.

C: No, I shouldn't think so. You will get adequate pain relief like everybody else.

RP: Thanks doc – you are not so bad. Maybe I will do something about getting off smack when I've had this abscess sorted.

C: That sounds like a good plan. I'm sure we can help you with it. Good day Mr Smith.

A more comprehensive drug history, which might include the patient's substance use over years previous treatment and so on, would not be expected during this brief assessment.

Sources

Department of Health (1999) *Drug Misuse and Dependence: Guidelines on Clinical Management.* London: HMSO.

Ghodse, A. H. (1995) Assessment. In *Drugs and Addictive Behaviour – A Guide to Treatment* (ed. A. H. Ghodse), pp. 120–147. Oxford: Blackwell Science.

Williams, H., Salter, M. & Ghodse, A. H. (1996) Management of the substance misuser on the general hospital ward. *British Journal of Clinical Practice,* **50**, 94–98.

Physical examination of a patient who has been drinking excessively

Construct

The candidate should demonstrate a professional, confident, caring and courteous approach to the physical examination of a patient with possible alcoholic liver disease. The candidate should exhibit due concern for the patient's comfort and dignity during the examination. The candidate should explain their actions to the patient as they go along for the examiner's benefit.

Instructions to candidate

You are a senior house officer who has been asked to admit Mr White, a 42-year-old publican with a long history of heavy drinking. Your consultant has asked you to note in particular any evidence of alcoholic liver disease. You have completed your history-taking and mental state examination and are now about to undertake a physical examination as part of the routine admission procedure.

Please examine the patient's head and neck, hands and abdomen in order to elicit any evidence of alcohol-related physical problems. Explain your actions to the patient as you go along for the benefit of the examiner. (Note that examination of the groin, genital and rectal areas is not required.)

Key points to be covered

- Introduce yourself to the patient and explain what you are going to do.
- When making the physical examination you should have regard for the patient's comfort and dignity.
- The specific areas of examination you have been asked to undertake are: inspection of head and neck, inspection and palpation of hands, inspection, palpation, percussion and auscultation of abdomen.
- You must provide an ongoing explanation of your actions to patient.
- You should give feedback to the patient when you have finished.

Suggested approach

- Introduce yourself, explain the nature of the examination to be carried out and try to put the patient at ease. Adopt a professional, caring and confident approach.
- Place the patient in a comfortable position for the examination (preferably lying flat, with one pillow under the head and hands by the side). Look before you palpate and always ask the patient about any areas of tenderness. Also, ask the patient to let you know if you hurt him at any time during the examination. Make sure your hands are warm and always palpate gently at first.
- Make a brief observation of the face and neck for evidence of jaundice, anaemia, spider naevi and so on, before going on to examining the hands and abdomen in more detail.
- Inspect the hands for evidence of palmar erythema, liver palms, clubbing, jaundice, bruising and Dupuytren's contracture.
- With regard to the examination of the abdomen, the patient should again be asked about any areas of tenderness and the examination should progress with inspection, palpation, percussion and auscultation.
- Inspection should note evidence of general swelling (e.g. ascites), dilated veins (c.g. caput Medusae), skin colour (e.g. jaundice, purpura) and so on.
- Palpation should include first a general, superficial palpation, followed by deeper palpation of the abdomen in general. You should then progress to specific palpation of the liver, spleen and kidneys. Remember when palpating the liver and spleen to start in the right lower quadrant.
- You should demonstrate the ability to percuss (e.g. the liver and spleen) and auscultate the abdomen (e.g. for bowel sounds).
- You should give feedback to the patient, especially with regard to negative findings, and thank him for his cooperation.

Sources

Munro, J. & Edwards, C. (eds) (2000) *MacLeod's Clinical Examination* (10th edn). Edinburgh: Churchill Livingstone.
Rubenstein, D., Bradley, J. & Wayne, D. (2002) *Lecture Notes on Clinical Medicine* (6th edn). Oxford: Blackwell Scientific.

Variation

A variation of this station could feature an intravenous drug user with suspected liver disease (e.g. chronic hepatitis). The examination would be similar to the one described for a patient who misuses alcohol, except that it would involve examination of the arms for evidence of injection marks, abscesses, cellulitis and so on.

Feedback on the results of investigations for alcohol misuse

Construct

The candidate should demonstrate familiarity with, and an understanding of, the investigations relevant to a history of alcohol excess, including the implications of abnormalities. The candidate is able to communicate these to the patient in a sensitive but honest manner, using appropriate opportunities to enhance motivation to change drinking behaviour.

Instructions to candidate

Mr Davies is a 40-year-old married decorator visiting you for his second psychiatric out-patient visit. He was originally referred by his GP, who thought he was depressed, but on his first visit you found a history of fluctuant dysthymia not amounting to a depressive episode and situational worries related to his business.

The history stretches back a year and seems to be related to problems with his decorating business, which is accumulating debt. You suspected he was minimising his reported alcohol consumption, although he did admit to drinking more as a result of the stress with his business, and you requested these routine investigations. He has come today asking for the results (shown in Table 8.1 – these would be available to you as a printout at the station).

Please discuss with Mr Davies the results of his investigations and their implications for his future health.

Key points to be covered

- An empathic, non-judgemental approach to the patient should be demonstrated.
- You should discuss the results in a non-technical, understandable manner with the patient.
- Be aware that no single investigation can identify alcohol use disorders with complete accuracy. Rather, these tests in combination with other clinical data can be seen as alerting factors.
- Relate the results in a non-confrontational manner and allow the patient opportunity for reflection and response.
- Try to link the abnormal results with the possibility of excess alcohol use. It may also be possible to relate some of the patient's presenting complaints to the consumption of alcohol.

Table 8.1 Results of Mr Davies' tests

Test	Result	Normal range
Sodium (mmol/l)	137	136–145
Potassium (mmol/l)	3.9	3.6–5.0
Urea (mmol/l)	5.8	2.0–7.8
Creatinine (mmol/l)	82	53–102
Albumin (g/l)	38	36–47
Alkaline phosphatase (IU/l)	103	36–126
Bilirubin (µmol/l)	12	2–22
Gamma glutamyl transferase (IU/l)	657	15–73
Alanine aminotransferase (IU/l)	44	5–36
Glucose (mmol/l)	3.7	3.9–6.9
Vitamin B12 (ng/l)	450	179–1132
Serum folate (ng/ml)	8.3	2.8–12.4
Haemoglobin (g/dl)	15.6	13–18
White blood cell count (10^9/l)	6.3	4–11
Platelets (10^9/l)	297	150–400
Mean corpuscular volume (fl)	102	79–98
International normalised ratio	1.0	0.91–1.06

- Feedback of test results can often serve as a powerful motivator for change for the patient. Biochemical tests also can be used to monitor clinical progress, and feedback of improvement in results may enhance motivation to maintain positive change.
- You should demonstrate a willingness to respond to any further questions from the patient.
- Follow-up arrangements should be confirmed.

Suggested approach

Opening

C: Hello, Mr Davies. My name is Dr —. I'd like to discuss with you the results of the blood tests that were taken on your last visit.

RP: Good. I've been a little worried about them.

C: Worried?

RP: Yes, in case they should show up something serious.

Follow-on

C: I should explain at the outset that blood tests like these rarely, if ever, are 100% certain of anything. Rather, when taken together with the story you have given us, they can sometimes be useful pointers to where problems might lie.

RP: I see. So how did I do?

C: I'm pleased to say that the vast majority of the blood test results were entirely normal. Two tests, the MCV and gamma GT, however, were a little outside the normal range. If you'd like to look here [it is useful to allow the patient to see the actual printout of the results] I'll try to explain. The first test, the MCV, measures the size of your red blood cells. In your case they are a little larger than usual. The gamma GT, on the other hand, is a test of liver function and it is also raised. It may imply that your liver is under strain or is working overtime.

RP: So what do you think is the cause?

C: There can be many reasons for the individual test results to be raised, but, as I said earlier, your other tests were all normal and you appear quite healthy. However, I do sometimes see this particular combination of a raised gamma GT and MCV in some patients who are drinking excessively. Would that make any sense to you?

RP: Well, yes, I suppose so. I did tell you I was under a lot of stress and perhaps I'd been drinking a little more than I've previously admitted.

C: So stress has been causing you to drink more?

RP: Yes.

C: Well, excessive drinking could certainly explain your test results and it might also explain some of the complaints you have been having, such as your anxiety and depressed mood.

RP: Does that mean my blood cells and liver are damaged permanently?

C: No, quite the opposite. If you can manage to reduce or stop your drinking, then you should see a steady improvement in these tests in the next few weeks or months.

RP: I would like to try to cut back on my drinking.

Closing

C: Why don't you keep a record of your actual drinking over the next couple of weeks? Then when we meet again we can discuss the various options available to you and plan how you might like to go about things.

Sources

Bien, H., Miller, W. & Tonigan, J. (1993) Brief interventions for alcohol problems: a review. *Addiction*, **88**, 315–335.

Miller, W. & Rollnick, S. (1991) *Motivational Interviewing: Preparing People to Change Addictive Behaviour.* New York: Guilford Press.

Variation: examination of a patient with suspected Korsakoff's syndrome

The scenario might centre on a 60-year-old, homeless street drinker who had been admitted a number of weeks earlier for alcoholic detoxification. The detoxification has been completed and the patient has been on no medication for 2 weeks. Nursing staff, however, note that the patient appears a little disorientated (for example he constantly loses his way around the ward) and to have a very poor memory. For such a station the instructions to the candidate might be 'As preparation for the weekly ward round, please carry out a cognitive assessment on this patient, with particular emphasis on his memory'. The assessment would be the same as that for the cognitive state examination in Chapter 7 (see pp. 63–65).

CHAPTER 9

Schizophrenia

Stephanie Young and Ranga Rao

Hallucinations

Construct

Candidates should demonstrate the ability to establish a rapport with the patient and be able to elicit hallucinations in a patient with psychosis.

Instructions to candidate

You are a senior house officer working in a general psychiatric ward assessing a new patient in the clinic. He is a 21-year-old man who has a 2-month history of social withdrawal, problems with sleep and concentration, and a decline in his academic functioning. There is also a history of personal decline. You have taken a history and have reached the point in the mental state examination where you need to elicit perceptual abnormalities.

Please elicit hallucinations.

Key points to be covered

- Establish rapport and introduce the topic of perceptual abnormalities tactfully.
- Elicit the form of any hallucinations, that is, their clarity, their relation to external objective space, the patient's volitional control over them, whether they occur in clear consciousness and the patient's insight into the phenomenon.
- Elicit the content of the hallucinations.
- Check for hallucinations that are part of the first-rank symptoms as well.

- Remember to check hallucinations in all modalities – auditory, visual, olfactory, gustatory and tactile.
- Explore risk issues.

Suggested approach

Opening

C: Could I now ask you something different, which we routinely check for completeness? Sometimes we have experiences where it appears as if someone is calling out our name and we turn around to find no one. Has this ever happened to you?

RP: Yes, I have had that on occasions and thought it was weird.

C: Could you tell me a bit more about it?

Follow-on

C: How clear were these voices?

RP: Well, they were pretty clear.

C: Would you say they were as clear as my voice?

RP: Yes.

C: Could you make out what they were saying?

Content

Explore whether these are true or pseudo-hallucinations or imagery. Does they appear to come from outside the patient's head? Can he stop them? Do they appear real? How many voices are there? What is the content of these? How did they refer to the patient – in the second or third person?

C: How do you cope with these?

RP: Well, I try not to concentrate on them.

C: Does that stop the voices?

RP: No, it doesn't. I have tried using headphones and playing music.

C: Does that make it better?

RP: Sometimes. I have also tried …

C: It must be distressing to have these voices constantly.

RP: I do sometimes feel I can't go on any more. …

C: Are you sometimes compelled to do what the voices have told you? Could you give me an example of a situation where you had to give in to the voices? Do the voices tell you to hurt yourself or others?

Closing

C: You have told me that you hear voices, which are clear, appear to be coming from outside, are distressing and sometimes ask you to do things. These have been going on for a few weeks and you also have had strange smells, which you can't explain. Even though you find it difficult to talk about them I am glad you have been able to share them with me. Is there anything else you wish to tell or ask me?

RP: No.

Sources

Wing, J. K., Cooper, J. E. & Sartorius, N. (1974) *Measurement and Classification of Psychiatric Symptoms: An Instruction Manual for the PSE and CATEGO Program.* Cambridge: Cambridge University Press.

Delusions

Construct

The candidate demonstrates the ability to establish a rapport and elicit delusions in a patient with psychosis and to explore the related risk issues.

Instructions to candidate

Mr da Silva, a 19-year-old man with a 3-month history of social withdrawal, has been referred to you by his GP. His parents have noticed that there has been a gradual decline in him socialising and he is more or less confined to his room. They have noticed that he is 'paranoid' at times. You have taken a brief history and have reached the stage in the mental state examination where you need to elicit any abnormalities in his thinking.

Please elicit delusions.

Key points to be covered

- Aim to establish a rapport and sensitively introduce the topic of abnormalities of thinking.
- Remember the patient may be guarded and not be forthcoming with information.
- Explore the content of his delusions while engaging the patient.
- Elicit the form of the delusions – evidence for the belief, ability to reason, sharing by subculture and how fixed they are.
- Remember to explore the related risk issues.
- Check for other delusions, such as delusions of reference, grandiosity, nihilism and so on.

Suggested approach

Opening

C: You were telling me that you've been a bit isolated recently and not going to college.

RP Yes. I've been feeling a bit depressed lately and trying not to go out.

Follow-on

C: Is there any other reason why you have not been going out lately?

RP: I guess I have not been too well and don't like going out much.

C: Sometimes people don't go out because they feel self-conscious in public; do you feel that is the case with you?

RP: Sometimes I do feel a bit uneasy when I go out.

C: Could you tell me a bit more about that?

RP: It is like I feel I am being followed.

Content

Explore evidence for the belief. Why does the patient think people want to harm him, and why him in particular?

C: So far you have told me that you feel that you are being followed by people whom you don't know, and you feel that this is part of a conspiracy. Is that right?

RP: Yes.

C: How long have you felt like this?

RP: For a few months now.

C: This feeling of there being a conspiracy to harm you – can I ask you how sure you are about this?

RP: Pretty sure.

C: If someone were to suggest hypothetically that they don't believe you, how would you respond?

RP: That is their problem, as far as I am concerned – this is what I am experiencing.

C: Would you mind if I ask you what your family's view is concerning this?

RP: I don't know. I don't think it they see it my way.

Closing

C: So far you have told me that you have been staying at home lately because you feel people are following you around and you feel that you may come to some harm as a result of a conspiracy. You have also told me about the other belief you have, about people talking and discussing and laughing behind your back. You don't know who these people are and even though you feel angry about this, you have not thought about doing anything in retaliation. Is there anything else you wish to tell me or to ask me?

RP: No.

Sources

Wing, J. K., Cooper, J. E. & Sartorius, N. (1974) *Measurement and Classification of Psychiatric Symptoms: An Instruction Manual for the PSE and CATEGO Program.* Cambridge: Cambridge University Press.

Negotiating a management plan with a patient who has been compulsorily admitted

Construct

The candidate is expected to communicate a proposed management plan to the patient, while maintaining the therapeutic relationship and allowing for a spirit of negotiation. The candidate should give the patient information about current mental state and adherence to treatment, while also preserving the patient's hope and minimising disappointment through an open and honest interaction.

Instructions to candidate

Miss Clinton is a 45-year-old single woman who was admitted to your ward 4 weeks ago, under compulsory detention for a relapse of her paranoid schizophrenia. She has now been stabilised on depot medication but does not believe that she suffers from a mental illness. She still needs great persuasion to have her depot injection and has residual psychotic symptoms despite considerable improvement. For the past week, Miss Clinton has been compliant with her 3 hours of unescorted leave from the ward to attend the local day centre.

Today it has been decided at the ward round that she is not yet ready for discharge despite her repeated requests, but she will be able to have extended periods of leave. She was told this in the ward round by the consultant but has not fully understood or accepted it, and is again asking to be discharged.

Please address her concerns.

Key points to be covered

- Explore whether there are any points that the patient had misunderstood at the ward round, as this may often resolve the problem.
- Assess whether it would in fact be possible to respect her request for discharge without compromising the overall quality of care.

- Even if these wishes cannot be agreed to, it is important that the patient is allowed to feel heard. This in itself may help to diffuse the situation and help to maintain the therapeutic relationship.
- If the patient is still in disagreement, remind her gently that an ongoing multifactorial approach continues to determine whether she is ready for discharge, with input from all relevant people involved in the care plan.
- Reiterate the rationale for not discharging Miss Clinton – her current mental state, insight, progress on the ward, adherence to medication and other treatments (e.g. leave from the ward), as well as risk – as this might help her understand the reasons for it.
- Although she needs to remain a compulsory in-patient, her increasing leave can be presented as a concrete step towards discharge and an indication of how well she is progressing.
- Finally, be empathic but do not make promises you cannot keep.

Suggested approach

Opening

C: Hello Miss Clinton. I've been told that you still want to be discharged home at the end of this week? Do you need some more explanation about what our plan was at the ward round?

RP: Well, quite frankly doctor, as I told you all, I feel much better and I want to get back to my own place. It's so dirty and noisy on the ward and I'm fed up with the food! But I'm still on this section ... can you get me off it?

Follow-on

C: I do understand your concerns. But the decision to remove the section is not just up to me. Everyone involved in your care discussed this today, and we felt you ought to remain in hospital. How do you feel now you've heard this?

Content

C: It's good that you no longer feel bothered by your neighbours, but you've told me that you still hear voices. We really want to get them to a level where you are no longer distressed by them. I'm also a bit concerned when you tell me you are not sure if you would continue with your injection if you went home.

RP: Well, if I get home, it must mean that I'm OK, so why should I have the injection?

C: Your injection is part of your treatment plan, and you might recall that when you were on tablets before you would not always remember to take them.

RP: Yes, but I am better now ... you give me leave off the ward and I always come back in time!

C: That's good but, as we explained, it can be stressful adjusting to being back home. That's why we've been giving you day leave, which we'll gradually increase to overnight leave in the first instance. That way we keep a close eye on how you're coping. Let's suppose you were to go home: how would you know if you were getting unwell again?

RP: I'm not sure what you mean doctor.

C: Well, can you think back to just before you came into hospital? Was there any change in the way you were feeling or anything different going on around you?

RP: Um ... the neighbours were annoying me and I couldn't sleep much because they were banging on my door all the time!

C: Yes, so maybe a change in your sleep pattern might be a sign of getting unwell, and knowing this means that we can give you the appropriate help.

RP: So, doc, does this mean that I can go home at the end of the week?

C: I have to be honest with you and say that we don't think you are quite ready to come off your section yet. We can give you more leave in the first instance, and it'll get formally reviewed at next week's ward round.

RP: I'm not happy about this! I want to speak to my solicitor! You can't lock me up any more! I'm well!

Closing

C: I hope you're not too disappointed with what I've said today, Miss Clinton. I do understand that you are keen to get back to your flat as soon as possible. It's been very useful talking like this and, as I said before, you are making steady progress. We'll keep reviewing the situation each day and take it from there.

Discussing the use of antipsychotic medication with a patient

Construct

The candidate demonstrates the ability to conduct a sensitive and propriately pitched discussion with the patient about starting suitable antipsychotic medication, and shows an awareness of the rationale, benefits and side-effects of such medication.

Instructions to candidate

You are seeing Mr Allen, a 25-year-old builder in your out-patient clinic. He describes a 2-month history of suspiciousness towards his family and colleagues, poor sleep and third-person auditory hallucinations. Mr Allen has been unable to work for the past month, but is keen to resume as soon as possible. He is willing to come back to see you for follow-up.

You decide to treat him for a first-episode psychosis and have explained the diagnosis to him.

Please now discuss the use of antipsychotic medication with the patient.

Key points to be covered

- Explore the patient's views, expectations and previous experience of medication.
- Avoid jargon as far as possible and pitch the discussion at a level appropriate to the patient.
- Tailor the choice and route of medication according to various factors, such as current environment (in-patient/out-patient), severity of current symptoms, duration of illness, number of relapses, insight, and previous adherence to medication.
- Explain common side-effects in a non-alarming but realistic manner.
- Explain that duration of treatment depends on multiple factors that are individual to the patient and to the nature of the illness.
- Provide reassurance that you will work with him to find the treatment that best suits him.
- If the patient seems reluctant to take medication, it can be helpful to use a motivational interviewing style to explore the benefits of medication, the likely impact on the patient's psychosocial functioning and the consequences of non-compliance.

Note that these points are equally relevant in other situations, for example, a patient who is due to start taking an antidepressant.

Suggested approach

Opening

C: Thank you for telling me about your recent experiences, which I understand have been distressing for you. Fortunately, there are good treatments for the symptoms you have, and in the first instance I would like to talk to you about the role of medication in this illness. Is that OK with you?

Follow-on

C: Mr Allen, I'm interested in knowing about what experience you have of taking medications in general, and also your initial thoughts on needing treatment for this illness.

RP: Well, I've only ever had to take painkillers for headaches in the past because I've always been a healthy person ... but I think I do need something to stop me feeling so tense. And these voices ... I know that I am not my normal self.

Content

C: You have described to me about feeling scared about people you normally get on with, as well as hearing voices. As I explained earlier, these are known as psychotic symptoms, and so the kind of medications we use are called antipsychotics. They work by correcting the chemical imbalance in the brain which is contributing to your illness. What are your thoughts about this?

RP: Hmm, I think I had an aunt who was a bit 'funny' in the head, and she had injections. ... I definitely don't want anything painful – I hate pain!

C: Yes, I do understand your concerns. The medication comes in a variety of forms, but we generally go for tablets or liquids that are swallowed, as it is the least intrusive method.

RP: Well, that sounds OK. How long does it take for these tablets to work?

C: There is no set amount of time, and it does depend on each individual, for example whether you get side-effects, or whether you remember to take your tablets. But in general, you could start getting some relief from your symptoms within 2 to 4 weeks, with even more improvement the longer you remain on them.

RP: What kind of side-effects might I get?

C: Well, first, not everyone will get them, and the good thing is that these new antipsychotics tend to have less troublesome ones compared to the older kinds. One of the most common side-effects is drowsiness. However, this is often minimised by starting off at a low dose, and taking your medication before you go to bed. In some cases being a bit drowsy is good, especially if you have problems sleeping or are otherwise feeling agitated. Other side-effects you might get are a dry mouth and increased appetite. However, these often improve over the course of the treatment, and many patients find that the benefits of the medication outweigh the side-effects. Of course, if at any time you feel you cannot tolerate your medication, we have the option of trying another one, which might suit you better.

RP: How long would I need to stay on the tablets?

C: Again, this depends on how your illness responds to the medication, but as this is your first time being ill in this way, we usually recommend staying on the treatment for 1 or 2 years after your acute symptoms resolve. In general, we do aim to give the smallest possible dose required to control the symptoms.

RP: But surely if I feel better I can stop the medication? It means I'm cured?

C: Please try not to stop your medication suddenly if you can help it. We know that patients can get unwell again even after recovering from their first episode of illness. Medication can be a protective factor in staying well, as well as avoiding other stresses, which we will also talk about later.

Closing

C: You've had to absorb a lot of information today, Mr Allen, and I'm really pleased that you have agreed to try — [medication]. If you have any further concerns about this treatment between now and our next appointment, please let one of the community team or your GP know. Also, you'll find some pamphlets at reception, which explain more about your medication. Feel free to take one.

Sources

National Institute for Clinical Excellence (2002) *Schizophrenia: Core Interventions in the Treatment and Management of Schizophrenia in Primary and Secondary Care*. London: NICE.

National Institute for Clinical Excellence (2002) *Guidance on the Use of the Newer (Atypical) Antipsychotic Drugs for the Treatment of Schizophrenia*. Technology Appraisal Guidance No. 43. London: NICE.

Spencer, E., Birchwood, M. & McGovern, D. (2001) Management of first-episode psychosis. *Advances in Psychiatric Treatment*, **7**, 133–140.

Explaining the diagnosis and prognosis of schizophrenia to a relative

Construct

The candidate demonstrates the ability to explain the aetiology, nature and course of schizophrenia to a relative in an empathetic, realistic and appropriately pitched manner, with some mention of both pharmacological and psychosocial treatments.

Instructions to candidate

You are with Mrs Dalton, the mother of a patient called Lisa, a 27-year-old shop assistant who was admitted informally to your ward 1 week ago for a 2-month history of auditory hallucinations, thought broadcast and suspiciousness towards others. She had had a similar episode last year which led to a compulsory admission, when Lisa improved on oral antipsychotic medication. She has no history of illicit drug use and was living with her boyfriend before this admission. She has now been restarted on atypical antipsychotic medication. Her mother has been worried about the implications of her daughter getting ill again and has arranged to speak to you about this.

Please explain the diagnosis and prognosis of schizophrenia to Mrs Dalton.

Key points to be covered

- It is important that information is tailored to the needs and concerns of the relative and that it helps reduce stress and the relative to cope with it. Avoid giving a textbook account of the illness, as it may be overwhelming. In the first explanation of the illness it may be better to give a general and realistic overview, but in a manner that instils hope.
- It may be useful to use a 'vulnerability–stress' model as a structure for discussion, and to outline: vulnerability factors that predispose an individual to developing schizophrenia; environmental factors (e.g. stressors) that influence the onset and course of symptoms; and protective factors, such as medication, stress management, social support and effective problem-solving tools. You need to be attentive to how receptive the relative is, and some of the information may be better given in subsequent meetings.

- When discussing prognosis, address the positive factors specific to the patient (e.g. previous adherence to medication, good social support) as well as factors that could be targeted to reduce the negative effects of the illness. Again, the amount of material conveyed must be in keeping with how responsive the relative is.
- It would be helpful to give the relative some theoretical knowledge of the prognosis, in order to provide a general indication of how the patient may get better or worse, and so on.
- Offer further opportunities for discussing the patient's care; you may also want to provide information leaflets that give the names of support groups and resource organisations.

Suggested approach

Opening

C: Thank you for coming here today Mrs Dalton. I'm Dr —, Lisa's ward doctor, and I understand you'd like to speak to me about your daughter.

Follow-on

RP: Yes, I'm very worried about what exactly is wrong with Lisa. She's normally a lovely, happy girl and it seems as if she's a different person now. I spoke to one of the nurses and she said Lisa has schizophrenia. That's really bad, isn't it?

C: Well, first of all, what do you understand by the term 'schizophrenia'?

RP: I've heard it's like being Dr Jekyll and Mr Hyde – a split personality?

Content

C: Many people have wrong ideas about schizophrenia. People with schizophrenia have one personality but may have problems distinguishing between what is real and not real. While some people with this illness may act in strange or irrational ways, more often they will behave quite normally most of the time.

RP: But I've read things in the newspaper where schizophrenics do horrible things – pushing complete strangers onto train tracks and the like!

C: Most people with schizophrenia are no more violent than people without the illness. Generally, they tend to be fearful of their experiences. Think of how frightened Lisa was when she first became ill.

RP: I suppose so, but what makes you so sure Lisa has schizophrenia?

C: Well, it is diagnosed when there are certain changes in thoughts, feelings and behaviours. For example, Lisa felt people could hear her thoughts being spoken out loud and was hearing voices, which is another sign of schizophrenia.

RP: What causes it then? Have I got 'bad' genes or something?

C: No, it is not your fault. The exact cause is not known but it's probably a combination of life stress and problems with the balance of chemicals in the brain. Stress can make the symptoms worse and possibly trigger the illness. Certain types of medication correct this imbalance.

RP: But I don't understand why Lisa got unwell again when she was taking her tablets. Didn't you say that medication gets rid of the illness?

C: Well, medication is just one factor, and I think Lisa wasn't always remembering to take her tablets. But even if you take your medication properly, you can still get unwell again, especially if you have a lot of stress going on in your life.

RP: Well, I just hope she'll be better soon. I have friends who own a shop and I was thinking of seeing whether they could give Lisa a job when she gets out of hospital. What do you think?

C: I think we need to see how Lisa manages day to day before making lots of plans for her.

RP: Alright then. Now, what about Lisa's medication? Once she's better and working she might not need it?

C: Although symptoms can be controlled with medication, as you have seen with Lisa we know that people are often more likely to get symptoms back if they stop taking it. We recommend that she stays on the tablets, but we may consider reducing the dose at some point in the future if she stays stable.

Closing

C: Mrs Dalton, I hope that I've been able to answer your questions about Lisa. I am aware that we have covered a lot of information today, so you might need some time to think it through. If you have further questions and concerns, I would be happy to arrange another time to see you again in the near future.

A routine out-patient follow-up review

Construct

The candidate demonstrates the ability to conduct a comprehensive out-patient follow-up on a patient who has now recovered from acute symptoms; the candidate focuses on mental state, relevant psychosocial factors, and medication efficacy, side-effects and compliance.

Instructions to candidate

You are in your out-patient clinic with Mr Brooks, a 31-year-old divorced man with a 4-year history of paranoid schizophrenia. He has been attending the clinic for the past 2 years. He has had several compulsory admissions to hospital for auditory hallucinations, paranoid ideation and self-neglect, but in the past 18 months he has been essentially stable on an atypical antipsychotic with regular input from his community psychiatric nurse (CPN), Tom. This is your first contact with the patient, who was seen by the previous senior house officer 3 months ago.

Please conduct a routine out-patient follow-up review.

Key points to be covered

- Establish a rapport and explain that you may need to go over parts of the history and treatment again, as this is your first time with the patient.
- Make a general assessment of current psychotic symptoms (if any) and screen for depressive symptoms. Do this if the patient is obviously well.
- Address any medication issues, such as side-effects and compliance.
- Enquire into the quality of the patient's engagement with community psychiatric services.
- Explore the patient's daily routine and assess any areas that could be improved. If you are unsure of how to address any of the patient's practical concerns, you could say that you need to find out who would be best to deal with them, rather than making immediate uninformed promises.
- Be empathetic in discussing stressors and other factors that could precipitate relapse – financial, housing, occupational or family issues (e.g. expressed emotion).

- Tactfully ask about the patient's use of illicit drugs and alcohol, as this may either precipitate or perpetuate the illness.
- Explore the patient's insight and awareness of early warning signs of relapse.
- It may be useful to structure your assessment as if you are doing a 'mini' Care Programme Approach review, bearing in mind the time limit and the need to be flexible, according to the patient's responses.

Suggested approach

Opening

C: Hello Mr Brooks. I'm Dr —. I've taken over from Dr —, who saw you at your last out-patient review. I realise that we haven't met before, so I apologise in advance if I need to ask you questions which you have talked through before. So, how have you been over the past few months?

Follow-on

C: I'm glad to hear that you are feeling OK. What do you think has helped?

RP: Well, I've been able to motivate myself more, especially now that I'm less slowed up since the medication was reduced last year.

C: That's great! What other differences has the medication made?

RP: I guess the voices haven't been around for some time now, and my concentration is much better. I'm even thinking of applying for a job as a security guard.

C: Oh, right. What enquiries have you made?

RP: I've sent off for some application forms but I'm not sure if I can fill them out properly ... plus I don't know how it will affect my benefits if I do get a job.

C: Yes, that can be a worry. I'm afraid I don't know the exact practicalities of these things, but perhaps your CPN could help you out. By the way, how are you getting on with him?

RP: We chat about what activities I could do during the day, but he's always asking me whether I'm taking my tablets. Winds me up a bit, sometimes.

C: I'm sure Tom is just concerned that you stay well; after all, he has known you for a long time now. I'm sure that you remember the difference medication made to you after coming into hospital?

RP: Yeah – I was less agitated and slept better.

Closing

C: It's been very nice meeting you, Mr Brooks. I'd like to see you again in 3 months' time. If you have any problems in the meantime, Tom is the best person to contact in the first instance. And as you are probably aware, I'll be writing to your GP about our meeting today and to ask her to keep prescribing your tablets.

Discharge from hospital to the community

Construct

The candidate is expected to be able to relate the care plan clearly to a stable patient who is ready to be discharged into the community. The discussion should focus on a 'bio-psychosocial approach', and cover aspects such as relapse prevention, crisis planning and adherence to medication, while giving the patient an opportunity to state his own goals and needs.

Instructions to candidate

You are the seniour house officer on the ward looking after Mr Ross Wilson, a 25-year-old man who was compulsorily admitted 2 months ago for a relapse of his schizophrenia. This was a consequence of his stopping medication, and disengaging with Sarah, his care coordinator. When he is unwell, Mr Wilson neglects his personal hygiene, eats less and believes that the Devil can speak to him. Occasionally he smokes cannabis, which tends to make his symptoms worse.

Fortunately, he has made a good recovery and has recommenced his antipsychotic medication. He was taken off his section at the beginning of the week and now it has been decided that he can be discharged back to his flat tomorrow. A formal Care Programme Approach review is due in 2 weeks' time.

Please discuss the issues concerning the discharge plan and follow-up with the patient.

Key points to be covered

- For this station it is suggested that you follow the format of a Care Programme Approach meeting on the eve of discharge. Therefore you need to be systematic in covering the biological, psychological and social needs of the patient. As there is often a lot of information to be covered, you need to ensure that you regularly check that the patient has understood what is being discussed.
- Explore the patient's views on what he thinks has helped the most in his recovery; for this, a motivational interviewing style might be helpful. You can highlight the factors which may be important to include within a relapse prevention plan. Also mention factors that might precipitate relapse, such as the use of illicit drugs.

- Discuss the importance of ongoing monitoring in the community and introduce the role of specific health professionals who will be available to review the patient. Explain the role of the care coordinator.
- Formulate a crisis and contingency plan, and explain it in a manner appropriate to the patient's understanding.
- Assess the patient's insight into and understanding of the need for medication and specifically agree who will provide and dispense the medication. Discuss potential side-effects.
- Address financial concerns, employment opportunities and accommodation in a sensitive manner, and always mention that you will refer to the appropriate professional if you are unsure.
- Ensure that you have made provisions for involving relevant family members in the discharge. In particular, a carer's assessment may also be needed.

Suggested approach

Opening

C: Well, it's good that you are now feeling ready to go home. What do you think has helped you the most in getting better?

RP: Being away from the neighbours, mostly. Also, getting back on medication – that's helped.

Follow-on

C: So, you have noticed a difference being back on your medication. I'm also glad that you aren't bothered by side-effects. I wonder how we can ensure that you continue to take your tablets? Do you have any ideas?

RP: I normally just take them out of that blue box.

C: Yes, that's your dosette box, but there were times in the past when you had difficulty remembering to take them. We'd be worried that if you weren't taking them for more than a week you might start hearing voices again. Sarah, your care coordinator, could support you if there are any issues to do with medication. What do you think?

Content

C: Right, let's talk about what to do if you begin to feel unwell again. It's important that we have a clear plan if this happens, so that we avoid getting to the point where you might need to come into hospital again. How would you know if you were becoming unwell again?

RP: I'd find it difficult to get to sleep.

C: Would you have any other problems?

RP: I suppose I wouldn't eat as well and would lose weight. ...

C: OK, that sounds reasonable: you don't look after yourself as well, hear voices, can't sleep and lose weight. Shall we say these are your early warning signs, which Sarah needs to look out for? If you or your family recognises these symptoms, Sarah would be the first port of call.

Closing

C: We've spoken about a lot of things today, Mr Wilson. All of them are important in helping you stay well once you leave hospital. We'll give you a copy of this in writing after your Care Programme Approach, and the ward staff can go through it with you again if you still have questions. I'll see you in 3 months' time, at out-patients.

Variations

Other OSCE stations that relate to patients with schizophrenia could ask the candidate to do any of the following:

- elicit a history of psychotic symptoms – the emphasis here would be on getting not only a good history of the present illness (mainly in terms of the psychotic symptoms) but also the relevant negative history;
- elicit psychotic symptoms – the focus here would be on the broad range of psychotic symptoms (i.e. delusions, hallucinations and first-rank symptoms);
- elicit first-rank symptoms;
- assess insight in the context of psychosis – here the emphasis would need to be on the broad range of measures that would indicate the level of insight, although views about the illness in general (apart from compliance issues and attitudes to hospital admission) could also be explored;
- assess risk in the context of psychotic symptoms – here the emphasis should be on risk to self and others, and the candidate would have to take care not to be drawn into simply elucidating the psychotic symptoms.

CHAPTER 10

Neurotic and affective disorders

Amrit Sachar

Mental state examination for mania

Construct

The candidate is expected to carry out a mental state examination of the patient, who is to be assessed for mood, biological symptoms, psychotic features and risk. The candidate is also expected both to establish a rapport and show empathy while interviewing the patient and to control the interview.

Instructions to candidate

You are an on-call senior house officer who has been asked to assess a patient in A&E by the casualty officer. The patient, Jennifer Marlowe, is a 29-year-old single mother of two young children, who has been brought to A&E by her sister. Most of the history has been obtained from the sister and she has told you that Jennifer has a 5-year history of bipolar affective disorder. She has had two previous formal admissions, both for manic relapses, but the patient has been stable on lithium for 2½ years. However, she stopped taking lithium a few weeks ago.

Her sister has noticed, in the past 2 weeks, that Jennifer has become increasingly irritable and impatient with the children and has also developed an interest in a number of new religions. Tonight, she announced that she was planning to go to India on a 6-week yoga retreat.

Please assess Jennifer's current mental state with specific reference to a possible relapse of her manic symptoms.

Key points to be covered

- You should be prepared, even before going into the cubicle, for a potentially difficult interview. While you are being assessed for the empathy you show, you are also being assessed on how well you control a difficult scenario.
- You will need to be fairly flexible during the assessment and may not be able to go through the mental state examination systematically.
- There may be parts of the assessment that you observe rather than ask about, such as the patient's appearance and behaviour, or the presence of pressure of speech. You can let the examiner know that you have picked up on these signs by saying, for example, 'I've noticed that you keep getting out of your chair' or 'It sounds like you can't get your words out quickly enough. Do you feel as though your thoughts come faster than you can express them?'
- When assessing mood and affect, remember to cover not only elation and irritability but also lability of affect, which may explain short episodes of low mood or even tearfulness. Ask about a few biological symptoms such as sleep, energy, interest and libido.
- Look for associated psychotic symptoms and if present establish whether they are mood congruent or incongruent.
- You may want to assess risk in the context of symptoms as you go along or separately.

Suggested approach

The focus of this station is on how to manage a difficult interview.

Opening

C: Hello Ms Marlowe. My name is Dr —. As you know, I've just been talking to your sister a little bit about what's been happening at home recently and she's been quite concerned about you. Were you aware that she's been worried?

RP: She's an interfering cow. She's got no right to be telling you stuff about me. She tricked me into coming here, you know. I know what her game is. She wants my kids. I bet she's told you a whole load of lies about me. And then you'll go off and tell a whole load of lies and so the story goes on and on and on, 'anon', 'upon', 'once upon a time ... there was a little girl called Jennifer .'.. You can call me Jennifer if you want.

Follow-on

C: Thank you Jennifer. You said that your sister's been telling lies?

RP: Lies, lies, lying. I was lying in bed and that's when it happened.

She injected me and now my children won't talk to me. They won't and don't and can't and shan't and ...

Content

C: Were you asleep at the time that she injected you, Jennifer?

RP: Of course. That *is* what people do in bed you know! Do you think I'm stupid or something? Do you think that I would let that cow inject me if I was awake? Man, you're just taking the piss. I haven't got time to talk to you. I've got things to do.

C: I'm sorry, Jennifer ...

RP: Don't call me Jennifer.

C: I'm sorry. The last thing I want to do is offend you and I certainly don't think you're stupid. I'm trying to get a better idea of how you have experienced the goings-on of the past few days. It sounds as if things may have been quite frightening for you and it feels as if you don't really know who you can trust.

RP: I can't trust anyone. Just myself. People always let you down.

C: In order that I can get a better idea of the situation, can you tell me why your sister would want to harm you or make you unhappy?

RP: Man, she's jealous of me, obviously. She wants me out of the way so she can be the greatest, but she'll never get rid of me 'cos I am the gre... well, I better not tell you.

C: Does it feel difficult to trust me?

RP: Well, yeah. I mean, what are you going to do with all this information?

C: I'm trying to find the best way to help you. I know in a lot of ways you feel very good at the moment, but it also seems as though you might be having some quite scary thoughts too. ...

Closing

C: Well, thank you for allowing me to have a chat with you. It has been very helpful to hear your side of the story.

RP: Yeah, but what are you going to do? You can't lock me up.

C: Well, I have to say that I am very worried about your safety and well-being. I'll need to talk to one of the other doctors to think about the best way for us to help you stay safe and improve some of the difficult experiences you're having at the moment.

Variation

- With a more stable patient, perhaps in an out-patient scenario, you may be asked to assess insight, in particular with a view to continuation of long-term prophylactic mood stabilisers. Remember that insight is not an all-or-nothing state. It varies from 'complete/full insight' to 'partial' to 'no insight'. It is important to explore whether the patient feels he or she has a chronic psychiatric illness, what may have contributed to relapses in the past, what has led to improvement, what the relapse indicators are and whether the patient feels the need for medication and follow-up to remain well. You would be expected to be able to relate to the patient some of the statistics about the likelihood of relapse if treatment is stopped.

History of anxiety

Construct

The candidate is expected to establish a rapport with the patient and show empathy while assessing her anxiety state; the assessment should include ruling out disorders such as panic disorder and agoraphobia, as well as the misuse of illicit or prescribed drugs or alcohol, and comorbidity (e.g. depression). Some assessment of the effect of the condition on the patient's ability to function and cope is expected.

Instructions to candidate

You are a senior house officer in a clinic seeing this patient for the first time. Her name is Mrs Shahnaz Khan and she is a 43-year-old married mother of two teenage children. She lives with her husband and children and works as a secretary but is currently on sick leave.

She was referred by her GP, who informed you that she has a 6-month history of worsening anxiety and panic attacks, and who has done tests to rule out thyroid and adrenal causes of anxiety. She has not been started on any medication.

Please take a history with regard to her anxiety.

Key points to be covered

- Remember that patients get very anxious about meeting a doctor for the first time and this will be particularly so if the patient is suffering from anxiety symptoms. If the role-player appears anxious in the interview, giving them feedback about this and using some simple distraction techniques or relaxation techniques may be helpful.
- Establish the criteria for a diagnosis. For example, is the anxiety generalised or episodic? If episodic, is it predictable

(phobia) or unpredictable (panic disorder)? Be aware that panic attacks occur in generalised anxiety disorder too, so establish whether there is anxiety between panic attacks. You need to look for a few autonomic symptoms but do not go through an exhaustive list.

- Establish the duration, onset and course of illness, as well as any exacerbating and relieving factors and triggers.
- Remember to assess the patient's use of drugs and alcohol. These not only can *cause* anxiety symptoms (e.g. amphetamines) and withdrawal symptoms (many substances) but also may be used by the patient as *a result of* the primary symptoms in an attempt to alleviate them. Do not forget prescribed drugs (e.g. benzo-diazepines) and evidence of dependence.
- Briefly rule out other illnesses such as depression, which may be comorbid or secondary to the anxiety.
- Get some idea about the effect of the anxiety disorder on the patient's functioning.

Suggested approach

Opening

C: Hello Mrs Khan. My name is Dr —. As you know, your GP referred you to us because she has been worried about you recently. I know you have probably gone through everything with her already, but would you mind going over it for me?

RP: Do I have to go over the whole story? I find it very difficult to concentrate.

C: It'd be helpful if you could tell me about the problems you've been having, in your own words, but there's no hurry. If we don't do it all today, we can finish next time.

RP: Alright. I'll try.

Follow-on

C: Your GP said in her letter that you've been feeling anxious and panicky. Can you tell me a bit more about that?

RP: It's been awful. It's taken over my life. I'm in a constant state of restlessness.

Content

C: And what effect does this constant restlessness have on you?

RP: I don't know really. I can't concentrate and I can't sit still for more than a couple of minutes at a time.

C: Are there any other physical symptoms you experience when you're feeling most anxious?

RP: Like what? I don't know what you mean.

C: Well, sometimes when people feel anxious or panicky, they can feel their heart beating really fast, or they get a dry mouth or feel quite sick. Do you get any of those feelings?

RP: Yes – I feel sick all the time. My stomach is constantly churning and sometimes I can't get my breath.

C: That must be quite frightening. Do you worry when you can't get your breath? [etc.]

C: So how long would you say you've been experiencing these feelings?

RP: Well, I've always been quite nervy, but it's just got so much worse in the past few months.

C: Do you know of anything that might have triggered it or anything that was happening at about that time?

Closing

C: Well, I'm afraid we're going to have to stop for today. Thank you for bearing with me. I know that it can be quite difficult at times to go through those questions, especially when you're not feeling well. But it was really helpful and it will allow me to get a better idea of how best to help you in the coming weeks and months. Have you got any questions for me?

Variations

- You may be asked to explain treatment options for anxiety, which would include problem-solving, distraction techniques, relaxation techniques, anxiety management groups, cognitive–behavioural therapy and medication such as selective serotonin reuptake inhibitors (SSRIs), selective noradrenaline reuptake inhibitors (SNRIs), or buspirone. Avoid benzodiazepines if possible and only use in the short term if necessary.

- You may be asked to try to establish the details of a first panic attack in taking a history of panic disorder. There is often a vivid recollection of this and it can be illuminating with regard to the psychological aetiology. Treatment choices are cognitive–behavioural therapy and a high-dose SSRI.

- You may be asked to take a history in relation to post-traumatic stress disorder, or to explain the diagnosis and its management. Familiarise yourself with the criteria for this disorder and the key features.

- If you are asked to explain the management of agoraphobia, the focus should be on communicating to a patient the cognitive–behavioural techniques and pharmacological treatments that may help.

History of deliberate self-harm

Construct

The candidate is expected to carry out a risk assessment, exploring whether mood disturbance, psychotic symptoms, alcohol or substance abuse have contributed to the episode of deliberate self-harm, while demonstrating empathy and an ability to establish a rapport with the patient.

Instructions to candidate

You are the on-call senior house officer in a busy district general hospital. It is early evening and you are asked to assess a 25-year-old man, Steve Jones, who arrived in A&E several hours ago after an overdose. He is presently unemployed and single – he split up with his long-term girlfriend a few months ago and has been finding it difficult to come to terms with this, especially as they have a 3-year-old son, whom he is missing very much.

He took an overdose of 16 paracetamol earlier today and was brought in by ambulance shortly afterwards. He has been medically cleared and has agreed to a psychiatric assessment.

Please assess risk in this man in the context of his overdose.

Key points to be covered

- Establish a good rapport with the client.
- Remember to be empathic and caring. You are more likely to get a good history from a patient whom you have taken care to put at ease. Do not allow the interview to sound like a checklist. Allow the patient to ask you questions and respond to the patient's cues.
- Even though you have been given some basic information about this man, you may find it necessary to go over some of it again with the patient, very much as you would do in A&E.
- Explore the *circumstances* of the overdose or the 'ABC of the overdose' (i.e. antecedents, behaviour and consequences). This includes whether the overdose was planned or impulsive: did he hoard tablets, were there any final acts (goodbye letters, wills), did he take drugs or alcohol with the overdose (disinhibiting factors), how was he discovered? Has he allowed medical treatment, how does he feel about the overdose now?
- Ask about any possible stress factors or precipitants.

- Assess whether there is any associated psychiatric illness, such as a mood disorder, psychotic illness or long-standing substance or alcohol misuse. Remember that you will not have time to go into the details of these. For depression, check a few of the biological symptoms and the negative cognitions of depression (worthlessness, helplessness, hopelessness).
- Look for any associated medical problems, such as chronic pain.
- Explore the likelihood of further acts of deliberate self-harm. His beliefs about himself and the world will affect this risk. How does he perceive the situation? Does he feel things can improve? Is he willing to engage with services? Remember that 'hopelessness' is highly correlated with completed suicide. You will also need to look at whether there have been previous attempts at self-harm, and the level of social support.

Suggested approach

Opening

C: Hello Mr Jones. I'm Dr —. I'm the on-call psychiatrist. Thank you for agreeing to see me. As you know, the casualty officer asked me to have a chat with you. I've been told a little bit about some of the problems you've been having recently. I understand this must be very difficult, but do you think you would be able to tell me about what happened yesterday?

RP: It's very embarrassing. I took some tablets. It's stupid really ...

C: Go on. ...

RP: What do you want to know?

Follow-on

C: Could you tell me a little bit about what it was that made you take the tablets?

RP: Well, I gave my boy, Davey, back to his mum, and I saw her with her new bloke. I suppose, until now, I always thought that there was still a chance that we might get back together. But yesterday it was as if that hope just disappeared.

Content

C: That must have been very upsetting for you.

RP: Yeah. I felt completely devastated all of a sudden and it was just, like, there's no point.

C: No point in what?

RP: Life, I suppose. It just felt like it wasn't worth it. What kind of a father can I be if I only see my son at weekends? I suppose it dawned on me that someone would take my place.

C: Where were you at the time that you started feeling like that?
RP: I was at home. There was no one in.
C: What had you done since you got home?
RP: Had a few beers and then thought about what tablets were in the bathroom cabinet.
C: Yes ...?
RP: I found a few paracetamols ... about 15 or 16. I'm not really sure how many.
C: Did you take anything else?
RP: No, just those ... actually, yes, there were a few of my mum's Valiums.
C: Do know how many?
RP: No.
C: You said a minute ago that you had a few beers. Do you remember how many? [etc.]

C: It sounds as if you've found things quite distressing since you and Jenny split up. How do you think this has affected your mood?
RP: I've been feeling quite depressed.
C: Would you say you feel like that most of the time?
P: These days, yes.
C: Sometimes when people get depressed, they find that they lose their energy. Have you noticed that?

Closing

C: That's been very helpful. Thank you for talking to me and I hope you didn't find that too distressing. Have you got any questions or is there anything you didn't understand?

Variations

- You could be asked to assess a woman with post-partum depressive symptoms. If so, you would have to explore the risk posed to herself and the baby. It would be important to look at aspects of the pregnancy, including whether it was planned, whether there were any problems in pregnancy, how she perceived the labour and whether there were any complications. Did the baby have to spend time in a special-care baby unit, or were there any other factors that may have disrupted the bonding process? Is she breast-feeding? If not, is that because she had difficulties with this? How does the health visitor think the baby is doing? Are social services involved? Does the baby cry a lot and how does the patient cope with this? You could enquire about the level of support that she receives, both practical and emotional, and about other children and previous pregnancies and postnatal problems. Last, you should explore whether there are any psychotic symptoms or signs.

- Alternatively, you could be asked to take a history of a patient with depression or do a mental state examination of a patient with depression, or to explain diagnosis and management to a patient or relative with a long history of bipolar illness.

History of obsessive–compulsive disorder

Construct

The candidate is expected to take a history in an empathic and sympathetic manner, in appropriately pitched language, to attempt to establish a diagnosis, and to rule out comorbid illness and substance or alcohol misuse. The candidate is also expected to explore the effects of the illness on the patient's life.

Instructions to candidate

You are a senior house officer in a clinic about to see a new referral. The patient's name is Andrew James and he is a 32-year-old single man who works as a computer analyst. The occupational health department at his company has referred him to you because of increasing concerns about his productivity and time-keeping. The occupational health physician, Dr Ellison, has already elicited some evidence of checking rituals and obsessive ruminations. She has asked for your help with diagnosis and management.

Please take a history of the patient's symptoms.

Key points to be covered

- Start with open questions, as always, and then move on to more specific questions about the compulsions and ruminations.
- The patient has been referred by an occupational health doctor, so clarify what the patient knows about the purpose of your session and also discuss confidentiality issues, as he may withhold information if he feels his job is at risk.
- Establish the diagnosis according to DSM–IV or ICD–10 criteria. In particular, you may need to probe quite a lot in order to differentiate between obsessive ruminations and delusional thoughts or passivity phenomena.
- Explore onset, triggers, duration, course, and exacerbating and relieving factors.
- Look for comorbid psychiatric illness. Remember that obsessive–compulsive symptoms can be a feature of other illnesses, such as

schizophrenia. It may also be that other illnesses have developed as a result of the obsessive–compulsive symptoms, such as depression.

- Screen for substance and alcohol misuse.
- Explore the effect of the symptoms on the patient's functioning. The information you have already been given indicates that there are problems at work. Look into these further and also ask about any effects on the patient's personal and social life.

Suggested approach

Opening

C: Hello Mr James. I'm Dr —. Thank you for coming to the clinic today. Before we start, can I ask what you know so far about this appointment or what you are expecting from today's session?

RP: Well, Dr Ellison said that some of the problems I've been having recently might be sort of psychiatric and that it would be worth seeing what you think.

C: That sounds about right. Dr Ellison has written to me asking for my opinion. She's told me a little bit about the problems and I will be attempting to look into those issues in a bit more detail today, so that we can figure out the best way to help. Now, it is important to say that, even though you were referred to us through your workplace, everything that we discuss is confidential unless you want me to feed back to them. Is that OK?

RP: That's fine. They've been really good at work. I'm happy for you to feed back to them and I've already signed a form saying that.

Follow-on

C: Alright. In your opinion, what have been the main problems recently?

RP: The main problem is that I've started falling behind at work. I have deadlines, which didn't ever used to be a problem and now I can't quite get on with things.

C: What do you think is the reason for that?

RP: Dr Ellison thinks it's obsessive–compulsive disorder.

C: OK. We can come back to what Dr Ellison thinks a little later, but it would be helpful for us to be able to discuss the actual symptoms you've been experiencing. What do you feel is keeping you from meeting deadlines?

Content

C: You mentioned earlier about having to check things. Can you tell me a little bit about what kind of things you're checking?

RP: That the cooker's off, the windows are locked and the taps are turned completely off.

C: How many times might you check these things?

RP: It used to be a few times but now it's seven times. It's a lucky number for me.

C: What do you feel would happen if you didn't check things seven times? [etc.]

C: You've already mentioned the difficulties that are occurring in terms of work. What other aspects of your life are being affected?

RP: I don't get to sleep until about 3 or 4 a.m. because of the rituals that I have to go through at night.

C: That must leave you pretty exhausted.

RP: Yes, it's awful. Then I can't get up as early as I need to in order to get them all done in the morning, so it just gets worse and worse.

C: And if you're so exhausted, what is the impact on your social and personal life?

RP: It's difficult to fit people into my schedule really.

C: What do your friends and family think about that?

Closing

C: Well, Mr James, we're out of time for today. Have you got any more questions you'd like to ask at this stage?

RP: Do you think I have obsessive–compulsive disorder?

C: This is only the first time that I have met you, and my assessment will be an ongoing process. But from the things that we've talked about today, there seem to be a number of features that would be in keeping with a diagnosis of obsessive–compulsive disorder. The positive thing is that it all started fairly recently and you seem to have a very good awareness of the problems. It's obviously having quite a distressing effect on your work and personal life, so it's important to start tackling the problems.

As it is a history-taking station, if the patient asks about management you will have to give only a *brief* reply – for example by offering to discuss it in more detail next time.

RP: How can I do that?

C: Well, we would do that together. There are tablets called SSRIs, which have been shown to be very good at improving the symptoms; psychological approaches have also been shown to be very good. Generally, using both approaches in tandem can have good results. We can discuss those in more detail next time and I can get you some leaflets about the medication and the psychotherapy.

RP: OK. That would be great.

C: Thank you for talking to me. Goodbye. See you next time.

Variation

- You could be asked to perform a mental state examination of a patient with obsessive–compulsive disorder, in which case you would be expected to focus on the nature of the psychopathology, to establish that the patient has obsessions and to go into some detail about the compulsive rituals.

Lithium and pregnancy

Construct

The candidate demonstrates the ability to discuss the risks and benefits of prophylactic lithium therapy in the context of pregnancy, while providing factual information and allowing the patient to make an informed choice.

Instructions to candidate

You are a senior house officer in a clinic seeing a long-term patient, Samantha Godfrey. She is a 27-year-old woman who has a 6-year history of bipolar affective disorder. Early in her illness, she was having one or two relapses per year, both depressive and hypomanic, and generally requiring informal admission. About 4 years ago, her insight and adherence to medication improved considerably, not least because of the influence of her boyfriend, Mark. In the past 4 years, she has taken lithium consistently and has had about one relapse every 2 years; during these she has been treated as an out-patient.

Today, she is euthymic and insightful, and tells you that she is managing very well in her current job (she works as a legal secretary). At the end of the interview, she tells you that she and Mark would like to start a family in the next year and wants to know what your advice would be.

Please discuss continuation of lithium in the context of her pregnancy.

Key points to be covered

- Sometimes an OSCE station involves a scenario that does not begin at the start of the consultation. As your ability to establish a rapport is likely to be examined for this station, it is still important to introduce yourself.
- Do not repeat the mental state examination if, as in this case, the instructions make it clear that it has already been completed. Use the information provided to take the interview on to the area that you have been asked to cover.
- Use an interactive, negotiating style, in which you provide truthful, easy-to-understand information, which allows the patient to make an informed decision about what is best. You can,

though, suggest which option you feel would be best and indicate why you feel this way.

- Start by finding out what the patient knows and build on that; dispell any misconceptions as you go along if necessary.
- Tailor the amount and depth of information that you provide according to: how well the patient is; the level of understanding the patient has; how much the patient wants to learn within a single session; and what stage of planning the pregnancy the couple are at (i.e. planning or just discovered that she is pregnant).
- Do not make the session sound like you are telling the patient everything you know about lithium in pregnancy. The skill is in judging how much to tell and how to tell it.
- Remember that there is no one right answer in cases like this one. This is a very good example of the need to carry out a 'cost–benefit' analysis, as there is no perfect solution.
- Discuss the risk factors for relapse – length of time on lithium, number of previous relapses, level of improvement between relapses, polytherapy and rapid discontinuation. Discuss the implication of a relapse, not just for the patient but also for the baby.
- Inform the patient of the risks to the foetus if she remains on lithium but also inform her of how this can be minimised.
- Outline the various options, such as coming off lithium slowly and monitoring mental state frequently, alternative medication or using the lowest effective dose.
- Mention other agencies that might help, such as the hospital's obstetrics department or perinatal liaison psychiatry service.
- End by offering the patient time to digest the information, provide reassurance that she can discuss these matters with you again and offer written information in the form of leaflets.

Suggested approach

Opening

C: Hello Ms Godfrey. I'm Dr —. I'm pleased to hear that things are going so well at the moment. And I'm pleased that you have come here today to discuss the options with regard to planning a pregnancy that will be as safe as possible for both you and the baby.

RP: Well, I remember you told me ages ago that I need to be really careful with contraception when I'm on lithium because it can harm the baby.

Follow-on

C: Yes, that's right, it can. I can tell you about the risks of staying on it during pregnancy and of coming off it, and then we can think about the best options for you personally. First, how soon are you hoping to start trying for a family?

RP: Soon. Sometime in the next few months if we get the go-ahead from you.

C: OK, so we need to start planning now really. We won't be able to cover everything in too much detail today, so I think it would be worth booking another appointment soon. We can get your boyfriend to come too and perhaps book a longer session. How does that sound?

RP: That would be helpful.

Content

C: What do you already know about the risks of lithium in pregnancy?

RP: I know that it can cause some sort of heart problems.

C: That's right. The main one is something called Ebstein's anomaly. It means that one of the valves in the baby's heart is not quite in the right place so it doesn't work properly. [etc.]

C: It is important for us to think about the chances of things going wrong if you aren't on lithium. It seems that you have been doing really well in the past few years.

RP: Do you think that's because of the lithium?

C: Since you've been taking it regularly, your relapses seem to have become less frequent and less severe, so it does certainly appear that it is stabilising your mood. What do you think?

Closing

C: We have discussed the benefits of staying on lithium and the way it might affect your baby if you stayed on it. I think you've probably had quite a lot to take in. We can arrange another appointment and I will give you some information leaflets. Do you have any questions?

RP: No. I will have to go away and think about our choices with my boyfriend.

C: OK. If you think of any questions, just write them down, ready for next time. It can all be quite confusing. Thank you for discussing all this with me.

Sources

Llewellyn, A., Stowe, Z. N. & Strader, J. R., Jr (1998) The use of lithium and management of women with bipolar disorder during pregnancy and lactation. *Journal of Clinical Psychiatry*, **59** (suppl. 6), 57–64.

Schou, M. (1990) Lithium treatment during pregnancy, delivery, and lactation: an update. *Journal of Clinical Psychiatry*, **51**, 410–413.

CHAPTER 11

Eating disorders

Rory O'Shea and Albert Michael

History of anorexia nervosa

Construct

The candidate demonstrates the ability to establish a rapport with the patient and take a history, looking in particular for symptoms of eating disorders, in a realistic and sensitive manner.

Instructions to candidate

You are a senior house officer in adult psychiatry. A GP has referred someone to your new-patient clinic. In the referral letter the GP states 'Please see Mary Kale, age 17 and currently doing A levels, living with mother (school principal), father (accountant) and 22-year-old sister. Tension headaches as a teenager, now has weight loss, diagnosis ?anorexia'. Her GP has ruled out physical problems leading to weight loss and endocrine causes.

Please take a history from Ms Kale. Ask about current symptoms of eating disorders and relevant aspects of the rest of her history.

Key points to be covered

- Establish a rapport and adopt a non-threatening manner.
- It is likely that the patient will be reluctant to attend, and this should be asked about and acknowledged.
- Enquire about the symptoms of anorexia nervosa (weight at least 15% below that expected; self-induced weight loss; body image distortion; evidence of hypothalamo-pituitary-gonadal axis dysfunction) and if present establish their duration.
- Similarly, symptoms of bulimia nervosa should be asked about.

- Rule out other mental illness, including mood disorder, anxiety disorder, obsessive–compulsive disorder and psychosis.
- Establish the patient's premorbid personality, mood, attitudes, values and interests, especially food-related ones.
- Explore the reasons for the patient presenting at this time.
- Take a family history – parents' and siblings' personalities and relationships with patient, plus family psychiatric history – as well as a personal history (relationships, academic ability) and medical history of the patient. (This may not be possible to cover in a 7-minute OSCE but it would be required as part of a comprehensive history of anorexia nervosa.)

Suggested approach

Opening

C: Hello Miss Kale. I am Dr —, the psychiatrist working here. [Shake hands.] Thanks for coming to see me.

RP: Hi.

C: As you know, your GP referred you here because he's concerned about your weight. I would like to ask you some questions about how you are feeling at the moment and about your background, to try to understand what is happening for you at this time. Is that okay?

RP: Yeah, fine.

C: Could I start by asking you how you how you felt about coming here today?

RP: I don't see why I should come here. I don't need to talk to anybody about what I eat. There's nothing wrong with me.

Follow-on

C: So you don't feel there is any reason for you to come here? OK. But your parents and your GP are worried about you.

RP: My mum worries only about how I do at school! My dad thinks I'm too thin. They both keep telling me to eat more.

Content

C: Can you tell me a little about what you eat?

RP: I just eat normal things.

C: For example, what did you have for breakfast today?

RP: I never eat breakfast. I work better without it. I usually have an apple at my 11 o'clock break.

C: OK, and what would you usually have for lunch?

RP: I always have two slices of crispbread and a Diet Coke.

C: Wow, I hate crispbread! Anyway, what's your next meal?

RP: Dinner. At dinner I have fish, vegetables ... whatever the rest of the family are having.

C: Do you have a family dinner together?

RP: No – I usually stay late at school for ballet or to study with my friend, so I have dinner on my own when I get in. It saves a lot of arguments too!

C: Arguments?

RP: You know, my mum telling me to eat, to do my homework, music practice, whatever. I'm not hungry usually. ... Sometimes I have a snack later but I'm trying to keep my weight down for my ballet – professional dancers are 50 kilos tops.

C: Oh, I see. Would you like to become a dancer?

RP: Yeah – either that or a lawyer.

C: You must be studying hard, trying to go to university?

RP: Yeah. ...

C: It sounds like you keep on a strict diet of low-fat foods to keep your weight down. I would like to know what else you do to keep slim. Do you exercise?

RP: Yes. There's my ballet class twice a week. I go to the gym for an hour and a half on Mondays, Wednesdays and Fridays, and I go swimming at the weekends. And I do 100 sit-ups every morning to keep my tummy flat. Britney Spears does 1000!

C: Really? She looks very fit ... but you look quite thin. Anyway, do you do anything else to keep your weight down? Have you ever taken slimming tablets?

RP: I sometimes take some fluid tablets that my Dad has if my weight is too high. But I don't take special slimming tablets.

C: What about laxatives, to make you go to the toilet?

RP: No.

C: Sometimes people make themselves vomit if they feel they have eaten too much. Have you done that?

RP: Yeah, sometimes, when I feel very fat.

C: How often do you make yourself sick?

RP   I've only done it three or four times ever!

C: What weight are you at the moment?

RP   Forty-six kilos.

C: Were you ever overweight?

RP: I was a bit overweight when I started at the school I'm in now and some of the other girls used call me names. But they don't any more.

C: Do you feel you are fat at the moment? Are there particular parts of you that you think look fat?

RP: I'm a kilo over what I want to be, which is a lot. My face looks okay but I hate my thighs – they are so fat and horrible – and my tummy looks fat and swollen too. I hate my thighs and my tummy.

C: I see. Can I ask you another question that might be a little bit embarrassing? It's about your periods ... what are they like?

RP: They don't come regularly. I haven't had one for 3 months now, and my last one was only for 2 days. They used to be regular up to about a year ago.

The other key points should be covered in a smiliar manner, if time allows.

Closing

C: OK, Mary. We have talked about your diet and eating habits, how you see yourself and how you keep your weight low. Is there anything else that you want to tell me or ask me?

RP: No.

C: I would like you to have some blood tests and see you again to get some details about your childhood and family. Is that alright?

RP: Yes.

Sources

Berg, K. M., Hurley, D. J., McSherry, J. A., *et al* (2002) *Eating Disorders: A Patient-Centred Approach.* Oxford: Radcliffe Medical Press.

Fairburn, C. & Brownell, K. D. (eds) (2001) *Eating Disorders and Obesity: A Comprehensive Handbook* (2nd edn), chs 48, 50 and 60. New York: Guilford Press.

Szmukler, G., Dare, C. & Treasure, J. (eds) (1995) *Handbook of Eating Disorders: Theory, Treatment and Research.* New York: Wiley.

Feedback of investigations to a patient with anorexia

Construct

The candidate discusses the results of blood tests with the patient and explains their significance in a sensitive manner using terms that the patient is likely to understand. Also required is an explanation of both the future course of treatment and further investigations.

Instructions to candidate

You are a senior house officer in a psychiatric out-patient clinic. You are reviewing a patient you saw for an initial assessment a week previously, at which time you diagnosed anorexia nervosa. The patient, Mary Kale, is a 17-year-old student who is significantly underweight, although she still feels she is fat. Her weight loss is a result of dieting, excessive exercise and sometimes self-induced vomiting.

Last week you took blood from Ms Kale. Today you have the results of the blood tests (urea and electrolytes), as shown in Table 11.1.

Explain the results and their significance to the patient and recommend further investigations and treatment, as appropriate.

Table 11.1 Ms Kale's blood test results

Test	Value	Normal range
Sodium (mmol/l)	129	132–144
Potassium (mmol/l)	3.0	3.3–4.7
Chloride (mmol/l)	95	95–107
Urea (mmol/l)	5.8	2.5–6.6
Creatinine (µmol/l)	73	55–150
Albumin (g/l)	29	36–47
Calcium (mmol/l)	2.06	2.12–2.62

Key points to be covered

- Check the patient's knowledge of these investigations.
- Use a motivational interviewing style.
- Give information in manageable amounts, checking that the patient understands (by asking her questions, etc.) and changing the pace of the interview and amount of information given accordingly.
- Adopt a sensitive, non-threatening manner, while emphasising the seriousness of the matter.
- Offer written information by way of leaflets and so on.
- Allow and encourage the patient to ask questions.
- Arrange to see her again, as there is a lot of information to pass on.
- Regarding the content of the investigations, you should advise the patient regarding:
  - hypokalaemia (the most acutely important abnormality) – its causes (vomiting, reduced fluid intake) and possible consequences, including cardiac arrhythmia (a common cause of death in people with eating disorders), intestinal dysmotility, skeletal muscle myopathy, neuropathy and chronic renal failure;
  - hypocalcaemia – can lead to osteoporosis and fractures;
  - hypoalbuminaemia – an important marker for poor nutrition and can lead to oedema;
  - hyponatraemia – can cause seizures and cardiac arrhythmias.
  - urea and creatinine currently normal – which indicates that there has been no renal damage – give a clear message to patient that it is relatively early in the course of her disease, that she needs to change her behaviour, and that it is not too late.
- Explain that further investigations are needed – such as a physical examination (if not already done), serum magnesium and phosphate,

full blood count, liver function tests, serum amylase, an electro-cardiogram, a repeat determination of urea and electrolytes, and also, in chronic cases, a bone mineral density scan.

- Tell the patient what she needs to do in order to get her blood test results back to normal.

Suggested approach

Opening

C: Hello Mary. Thank you for coming back to see me. How have you been since last week?

RP: OK.

C: Good. The results of your blood tests are back. Would you like to know what they are like?

RP: Yes please.

Follow-on

C: First, can I ask you why you think we requested these tests?

RP: I suppose you wanted to see if my eating pattern has caused any changes in the blood, like dehydration.

C: You are right. There are certain changes in your blood [shows patient the report, reproduced here as Table 11.1]. The sodium, potassium, chloride and calcium are salts in your blood. The number beside each tells you how much of each you have in your blood. The next column of numbers shows how much you should have. And as you can see, there are some numbers that are below the normal level.

RP: What does this mean?

C: This means that you don't have enough of these in your blood.

Content

RP: Do you know what causes this?

C: The most likely causes of these changes are vomiting and not eating or drinking enough. You take in these salts when you eat or drink but they are lost from your body when you vomit.

RP: I suppose I was inducing vomiting and also using laxatives. Do you think it is dangerous to have too little of these salts?

C: Your results are not too bad at the moment, but if they got worse it could be very dangerous. The one that can be most serious is the potassium. When it gets too low it affects your heart – your heart beats too fast or beats irregularly, and that can cause a kind of heart attack.

RP: I thought only fat old people get heart attacks.

C: People your age can too, I'm afraid. It's the most common cause of death in people with anorexia. Low potassium can also damage your muscles, stop your tummy and gut from working properly and eventually damage your nerves and kidneys very badly.

RP: So you're saying I'm going to die?

C: No, I don't think so, Mary. I know you are very worried, but your results are not too bad at the moment – they are not dangerously low.

RP: How can I get them back to normal?

C: The most important thing is for you to eat a healthier diet and try to stop making yourself sick. We can offer you advice on this and refer you to a dietician. In the meantime I will prescribe some potassium tablets for you to take twice a day.

Similar explanations should be given for the other abnormalities, as far as time allows. If running out of time, the candidate should:

- explain that time is limited and apologise for this
- offer to see the patient again
- concentrate on the key points
- if all key points have not been covered, mention them during the 'closing', as points to be coverd in the next interview.

Closing

C: To summarise, we have been discussing the results of your blood tests, what they mean and ways of getting them back to normal. We may also need to do further tests. Do have you any questions?

RP: No.

C: Could I give you these leaflets to read and maybe arrange to see you again in 2 weeks' time? If you have any questions on what we have discussed, you can ask them then, as it might be a lot to take in today.

RP: Thank you doctor.

Sources

Freeman, C. P. L. (1998) Eating disorders. In *Companion to Psychiatric Studies* (6th edn) (eds E. C. Johnstone, C. P. L. Freeman & A. K. Zealley), pp. 509–528. Edinburgh: Churchill Livingstone.

Halmi, K. A. (2001) Physiology of anorexia nervosa and bulimia nervosa. In *Eating Disorders and Obesity: A Comprehensive Handbook* (2nd edn) (eds C. Fairburn & K. D. Brownel), pp. 267–271. New York: Guilford Press.

Kaplan, A. S. & Garfinkel, P. E. (eds) (1993) *Medical Issues and Eating Disorders: The Interface.* New York: Brunner/Mazel.

Sharp, C. W. & Freeman, C. P. L. (1993) The medical complications of anorexia nervosa. *British Journal of Psychiatry*, **162**, 452–462.

Explain the diagnosis and prognosis of anorexia nervosa to a relative

Construct

The candidate is expected to establish a rapport with a patient's relative, and to discuss the diagnosis and prognosis of anorexia nervosa in a sensitive manner, pitched appropriately to the level of understanding of the relative, while conveying factual information and clarifying any misconceptions.

Instructions to candidate

A 17-year-old woman, Mary Kale, has recently been admitted under your care. You have made a diagnosis of anorexia nervosa, based on her history (of weight loss, dieting, excessive exercising, body image distortion and amenorrhoea) and investigations. Her father has difficulty accepting the diagnosis.

Please discuss with him the diagnosis and explain the likely prognosis.

Key points to be covered

- Introduce yourself, shake hands, thank him for attending and explain how much time you have.
- Use language appropriate to his level of comprehension (i.e. do not confuse him with technical terms or patronise him).
- Be sensitive, especially when imparting distressing information such as mortality figures.
- Assess his baseline knowledge of the reasons for his daughter's hospital admission, and his view of the nature of his daughter's problems and current difficulties.
- Use that information to build up a set of core symptoms of anorexia nervosa and introduce the diagnosis. Assess his response to this.
- Address any misconceptions.
- Deal empathetically with any emotional responses to the diagnosis.
- Give the overall prognosis for anorexia nervosa. This is very variable. A summary of the literature is that after 10-year follow-up 50% had no eating disorder, 15% had a subthreshold eating disorder, 15% had developed bulimia nervosa, 10% had persisting anorexia nervosa and 10% were dead. Patients with eating disorders are more likely to have affective disorders and anxiety disorders.

- Discuss positive and negative prognostic factors as they relate to the patient. Poor prognostic indicators are older age at onset, premorbid obesity, long duration of illness before treatment, personality disturbance, bulimic symptoms, male gender and short treatment follow-up.
- Discuss briefly how treatment can improve the likely outcome.
- Summarise at the end, offer written information and arrange to meet again for a further session to clarify.

Suggested approach

Opening

C: Hello Mr Kale, I'm Dr —. I'm glad you could attend this appointment to talk about what might be going on with Mary.

RP: Thanks for your time.

Follow-on

C: Mr Kale, we have about 7 minutes. I'd like to start by asking you some questions, and then you can ask me anything that's on your mind. Is that all right?

RP: That's fine.

C: Great. I have been speaking to your daughter, obviously, and to your wife, but not to yourself before now. Tell me, do you feel Mary has any problems at the moment?

RP: As you know, she has not been eating much and is losing weight.

Content

C: Do you think there's anything wrong with her eating? Do you see her as underweight?

Further questions could include 'What do you think could be causing all of this?', 'Does she agree?', 'Do you think her weight is dangerously low?', 'What does she do to keep her weight down?' It may be inappropriate to ask the father about amenorrhoea.

C: Based on the information you have given and the tests we have done [it may be appropriate here to summarise the key facts], it appears that she may have a condition called anorexia nervosa. Have you heard of it?

RP: I have heard that it is a condition that affects young girls and could be fatal.

C: What else do you know about this?

RP: They do not eat and starve themselves and have problems. Do you think Mary is suffering from this?

C: As I was saying, she has many of the key features and unfortunately it appears to be the most probable diagnosis at this stage. The main features are … and, as you were saying, she has these.

RP: Is it possible she may have another illness?

C: As you are aware, we have examined her and have done tests to rule out any other conditions. ...

RP: What happens to patients with anorexia? Do they get better?

C: It is variable and depends on the response to treatment. ... [Give an overview of the factual information regarding the prognosis.]

C: In terms of her treatment we can offer the following ...

Closing

C: We have briefly discussed your daughter's illness, treatment options and what happens if the condition is not treated early. It might be too much information to take in at once and maybe we need to meet again to discuss it in more detail. Here are some leaflets on anorexia nervosa. Do you have any questions?

RP: Let me go through the stuff you have given me and I will come back to you.

Sources

Steinhausen, H. (2002) The outcome of anorexia nervosa in the 20th century. *American Journal of Psychiatry*, **159**, 1284–1293.

Sullivan, P. F. (2001) Course and outcome of anorexia nervosa and bulimia nervosa. In *Eating Disorders and Obesity: A Comprehensive Handbook* (2nd edn) (eds C. Fairburn & K. D. Brownell), pp. 226–230. New York: Guilford Press.

Szmukler, G. I. & Russell, G. F. M. (1986) Outcome and prognosis of anorexia nervosa. In *Handbook of Eating Disorders: Physiology, Psychology and Treatment of Obesity, Anorexia and Bulimia* (eds K. D. Brownell & J. P. Goreyt). New York: Basic Books.

History of bulimia nervosa

Construct

The candidate demonstrates the ability to take a history in the context of symptoms of bulimia nervosa, while being able to rule out differential diagnoses.

Instructions to candidate

As a senior house officer in psychiatry, you are asked to see Miss Barker, a 23-year-old bank clerk, in the out-patient clinic. Her GP, who has referred her, says that she has insulin-dependent diabetes mellitus and he has recently become concerned about her diabetes control. She has told him she has been omitting her insulin in order to lose weight. She has said that she makes herself vomit when she feels that she has eaten too much.

Please take a history in the context of an eating disorder.

Key points to be covered

- Perform the interview in a sympathetic, non-threatening manner (as the patient may be anxious and is likely to be embarrassed about her problem).
- Observe the general principles of interviewing for history-taking, such as the use of open-ended questions, facilitation, summarising and feedback at regular intervals.
- Aim to establish a rapport and demonstrate empathy.
- Ask about the key symptoms of bulimia nervosa:
  - persistent preoccupation with eating, and irresistible craving for food, leading to episodes of overeating in which large quantities of food are consumed in short periods of time;
  - attempts to counteract the fattening effects of food by one or more of the following: self-induced vomiting; misuse of purgatives; periods of starvation; use of drugs (appetite suppressants, thyroid drugs, diuretics, neglect of insulin treatment for diabetes);
  - a morbid dread of fatness.
- Explore precipitating, predisposing and maintaining factors.
- Rule out differential diagnoses such as anorexia nervosa, depressive illness, obsessive–compulsive disorder and overeating associated with other psychological disturbances.
- Report your key findings to the patient at the end, offer a provisional diagnosis and assess her opinion of your diagnosis (i.e. her insight).

Suggested approach

Opening

C: Hello, I am Dr —. Thank you for coming to see me.

RP: Hello.

C: Miss Daily, your GP has become a bit worried about your blood sugar level – it has been running quite high, I think?

RP: Yes. Well, sometimes.

Follow-on

C: I would like to ask you some questions about your diabetes and about your eating habits, as well as how you are feeling in yourself, things like that – just to see if you think you have any problem with your diet and so on, and whether I can help you with anything. Is that all right?

RP: Yes.

Content

C: Can I start by asking you if you feel you have any problems or difficulties at the moment?

RP: I am trying to lose weight, and I know that if I don't take so much insulin my weight will go down.

C: Could you tell me a bit more about that?

RP: So sometimes I don't take the right amount of insulin ... if I weigh myself and find that I've put on weight, I take less insulin for a few days so that my weight goes down.

C: I see. Please go on.

RP: There are times when I eat a lot and then feel guilty about it....

C: What happens next?

RP: Sometimes I make myself vomit so that I don't get fat. But then I feel even worse, like I'm not in control of myself. Then I feel really sad and start crying and thinking I'm terrible. I am terrible – I can't control my eating! ...

C: I'm sorry you feel so bad sometimes. I hope that we can help you to be more in control of yourself and feel better about yourself. So far you have told me that you tend to eat a lot in binges and then induce vomiting. You have also used purgatives in order to lose weight but have not used any other drugs. Could I ask you what triggers these binges?

RP: Usually it is when ...

C: Can I ask you what you think about yourself compared to other people?

RP: I think I am ugly and fat. I'm not very confident. I don't really like myself.

Closing

C: Ms Barker, so far you have told me about your problem with weight and eating, that you have not lost significant weight and that your periods are normal. However, it is interfering significantly with your diabetes. Is there anything you would like to tell me or ask me?

RP: What do you think is wrong with me?

C: Well, based on what we have been discussing, you appear to have many of the symptoms of bulimia. I will tell you more about bulimia and give you some information to read so that we can discuss this when you see me next.

RP : Thank you.

Sources

Beumont, P. J. V. (2001) Clinical presentation of anorexia nervosa and bulimia nervosa. In *Eating Disorders and Obesity: A Comprehensive Handbook* (2nd edn) (eds C. Fairburn & K. D. Brownell), pp. 162–170. New York: Guilford Press.

Garfinkel, P. E. (2001) Classification and diagnosis of eating disorders. In *Eating Disorders and Obesity: A Comprehensive Handbook* (2nd edn) (eds C. Fairburn & K. D. Brownell), pp. 155–161. New York: Guilford Press.

CHAPTER 12

Psychosexual disorders

Nick Dunn

Assessment of erectile dysfunction

Construct

The candidate engages the patient and establishes that the patient has erectile dysfunction, as distinct from premature ejaculation. The candidate should assess possible causes, such as any drugs taken and general health. The effect on his relationship needs to be appropriately explored.

Instructions to candidate

Dear Dr —
Regarding Mr R Booth
23 Witham Street
Forest Hill
Manchester

I would be grateful for your help with Mr Booth, a long standing patient of mine. He is 67 years old. His wife died 5 years ago and he has started a relationship with a woman who is 50. He complains that his erections are unsustained and this is causing concern to them both. I doubt that she will be present for the interview as she has told me that the problem is clearly his.
His medication is unchanged for years:

- aspirin one tablet daily – he suffered a transient ischaemic attack 2 years ago;
- bendrofluazide – he has been taking this for over 15 years.

Yours sincerely
Dr Gupta
General Practitioner

Please take a history in the context of this patient's erectile dysfunction.

Key points to be covered

- Establish a rapport.
- Assess the patient's pattern of erectile dysfunction.
- Explore its effect on social functioning and relationships.
- Check for interactions with any medication and exclude hypertension and diabetes.
- Ask the patient about any treatments tried so far.
- Establish his view of his erectile dysfunction and what he thinks would lead to improvement.
- Ask about the attitude of his partner to him wanting a sexual relationship.
- Introduce the idea of a rating scale to monitor progress.
- Discuss self-help and education.

Suggested approach

Opening

C: Your general practitioner has written explaining your difficulties with erections. Is that what you're having?

RP: Yes.

C: I will need to ask you some questions about this – about how it started, and how it has affected you. Is that OK?

RP: That is why I'm here.

Follow-on

C: Was there a time when your erections were normal?

RP: Yes, when my wife was alive, about 5 years ago.

C: Since then have you had an erection?

RP: Well, I have not had a partner.

C: What about an erection in the morning?

RP: Yes they still happen.

C: And at night?

RP: No, I can't remember those.

Content

C: Can you get an erection by yourself?

RP: Yes, I could.

C: So tell me, what happens when you try to get an erection with your partner?

RP: It just will not last and then both of us are disappointed.

C: Do you ejaculate before you lose the erection?

RP: No.

C: It sounds like your erections are better without your partner present. Would that be right?

RP: Yes. It's as if Jane, my partner, makes me nervous.

C: How have you both coped with this?

RP: Well, she says that it does not matter, but she is a young woman and will find contentment elsewhere unless I can sort this out.

C: What treatments have you tried so far?

RP: None. My partner wanted me to try Viagra off the internet, but I think it is dangerous to dabble with drugs without a doctor involved.

C: Does your partner know that you are coming to this clinic?

RP: Yes. She wanted to come as well but I thought I would check it out by myself first.

C: Sounds like she is keen to get things sorted. Do you feel under pressure?

RP: Yes. She seems in such a hurry.

C: Why do you think this has happened to you?

RP: In a nutshell, I think Jane thinks I want sex more than I do – or I think she wants it more than me. Anyway, it gets me thinking about it, and worrying that it is not going to last and, yes, that is exactly what happens.

Closing

C: How would you feel about Jane coming with you next time?

RP: OK, now I know what kind of questions you ask.

C: In the meantime, would you fill in this questionnaire so I can have some idea about where you are now and so that your progress can be monitored?

RP: OK. Is there anything else you would like me to do before next time?

C: Yes, you can read this book on male sexual problems and perhaps next time we can discuss what you think of it.

Sources

Andrews, G. & Jenkins, R. (eds) (1999) *Management of Mental Disorders* (UK edn). Sydney: World Health Organization Collaborating Centre for Mental Health and Substance Abuse.

Assessment of loss of sexual interest in a woman

Construct

The candidate must demonstrate the ability to gain a rapport with and engage the patient, take a brief history that discriminates primary from secondary loss of arousal, and explore the interaction with the contextual factors of the general relationship and any medical and social problems.

Instructions to candidate

Dear Dr —

Mrs Forshaw

This mother of two pre-school children complains of loss of sexual interest. All endocrine blood levels are normal and her two lively boys are healthy. Her husband is an NHS manager who has recently been promoted. I would be grateful if she could be assessed by your service.

Yours sincerely

Dr Tom Kalafatis

General Practitioner

Please take a relevant history in the context of loss of sexual interest.

Key points to be covered

- Demonstrate an empathic style and be alert to the emotions expressed by the patient.
- The assessment must cover the patient's psychological state in the context of her marital relationship.
- Any changes in her presenting complaint must be correlated with changes in her psychological, social and relationship domains, particularly the effect of children on her relationship.
- Assess her attitudes to sex, her knowledge about sexual matters, her general relationship, her self-esteem and any history of sexual trauma.
- The response of the patient's partner to the difficulty needs exploration.
- Key factors that distinguish between primary and secondary loss of arousal are whether there was a period of normal sexual

functioning before loss of arousal (secondary) or whether things have always been this way (primary).

Suggested approach

Opening

C: Hello, my name is Dr —. Your GP, Dr Kalafatis, has written asking me to help you with a sexual difficulty. Is that your understanding of why you are here?

Follow-on

RP: Yes. We used to have a pretty normal sexual relationship, but now I just never seem to be in the mood. It is upsetting us both. I wish I could turn back the clock.

C: Sounds as though things were fine, then they stopped being fine. Is it possible to say when that happened?

Content

RP: I think it was after the birth of our second child. He was a poor sleeper and feeder. I just seemed permanently exhausted. That is roughly when I kind of lost interest.

C: And are you still exhausted?

RP: No, not at all. It's just that sex has crept off my mental agenda. We expected it to come back but it didn't.

C: Can you enjoy other things like you used to?

RP: Yes – I enjoy the two boys and we go out together. They do have a habit of coming into our bedroom at night, though.

C: And do you and your husband miss the loss of privacy?

RP: Well, they are company, you see. My husband is often late and rather stressed out by his work. Even when he is home he has loads of e-mails to get through

C: Are you saying that there is less time for sex nowadays?

RP: Most definitely. It is all a rush.

C: When you are on holiday does your libido return?

RP: Libido?

C: Your sex drive.

RP: You would think it would but it has not.

C: When you were last on holiday did you have more time to relax?

RP: It was not really a holiday, as my husband assumed my sex drive would snap back and, to be truthful, so did I. It was a huge disappointment to him.

C: How has your husband coped with this change in you?

RP: He thought I was going off him and started buying me lots of presents. He's rather gone into overdrive as compensation I suppose.

C: How is your general health?

RP: Good I would say. My GP did a lot of tests but they were all normal.

Closing

C: So, in summary, it seems you had a normal sex life before your second child. The loss of sex drive seemed to be at roughly the same time as your period of exhaustion, and then despite getting your energy back your sex drive has not returned, even on holiday. Your husband is pressured at work and has less time for you and if anything he has tried initiating sex more often than before.

History-taking from a patient experiencing premature ejaculation

Construct

The candidate engages the patient and establishes that the patient has premature ejaculation rather than erectile dysfunction, while exploring the aetiology and any effect on relationships.

Instructions to candidate

Dear Dr —

Re: Mr Martin Smith
The Bunkers
Chipping Mews
London SW1

Thank you for seeing Mr Smith. He is golf secretary at the local course. Mr Smith complains of premature ejaculation. He is about to marry Lisa, a barmaid who works at the same golf club; he is worried about how he will survive the honeymoon. They make a rather incongruous couple in that he is totally devoted to golf and etiquette at the club, and she seems to be wanting to marry and have a family. She was married before, although for only 2 years. I have checked his blood pressure, which is within normal limits, and his fasting blood sugar is within normal range.

Dr Tom Durcan

General Practitioner

Please take a history in the context of his premature ejaculation.

Key points to be covered

- Establish a rapport and engage the client.
- Establish the diagnosis of premature ejaculation by eliciting onset, pattern and pervasiveness. Clarify the frequency of masturbation and intercourse, and whether control over ejaculation is easier with masturbation than intercourse (if so, determine for how long can that control be maintained).
- If avoidance of sexual behaviour is suggested, then this should be tactfully addressed.
- Enquire about the effect of the problem on social functioning, the relationship, the partner's response to this problem and her views on the sexual relationship.
- Explore possible interactions with any medication.
- Exclude hypertension and diabetes if this has not been done by the patient's GP.
- What treatments has the patient tried to delay ejaculation?
- Establish the patient's view of his premature ejaculation and what he thinks would lead to improvement.
- Introduce the idea of a rating scale to monitor progress.
- Discuss self-help and education.

Suggested approach

Opening

C: Your general practitioner has written explaining that you are having difficulties with your sexual relationship. Is it OK to talk about this?

RP: Yes, that's what I want to sort out.

C: I will need to ask you some questions about this – about how it started, and how it has affected you. Is that OK?

RP: That is why I'm here.

Follow-on

C: Was there a time when your sexual performance was in your view satisfactory?

RP: That is difficult to say because I think I came to sex rather late in life.

C: How old were you when you became aware of sexual matters?

RP: I was a virgin until 35, if that is what you mean.

C: Not really. Most children growing up experience sexual matters educationally from school or parents.

RP: My parents, no, they would not talk about it – but it was discussed in biology classes at school. But sex-wise I have never played to par.

C: How old were you when you started to masturbate?

RP: I didn't really. I was aware the other boys were doing it at school but I could not see the point – never have. I was more into sports you see – golf, tennis, cricket, anything like that.

C: What there anything that put you off?

RP: What, sport? No, never. Loved it. It is my life really.

C: No, I am talking about masturbation. Was there anything that worried you about masturbating during adolescence?

RP: I thought that I ought to save myself for the person I was to marry.

C: I understand you are going to marry soon.

RP: Yes. She is a bit keener on the sex side of things than me, and we have attempted it a few times.

C: Are you able to say what happened?

RP: Yes. I became overexcited and it was all over before anything started at all. Like rushing the back swing. She was not happy. I think that she is more experienced than me. She was married, you know.

C: Did you tell her that you were saving yourself for her?

RP: Yes – she thought it was ridiculous! She didn't like the idea that she was going to have to teach me everything. Mind you, I don't like playing golf with a complete beginner myself – very slow and they don't know how to manage themselves on the course. Do you play golf?

C: It sounds like you feel a complete beginner when it comes to sex with Lisa. Has this led to disagreements or even rows?

RP: She was the one that suggested that I go to my doctor. She has scoured the internet for treatments. She wanted to come here with me but I preferred to see you alone first.

C: What treatments have you tried so far?

Closing

C: How would you feel about Lisa coming with you next time?

RP: OK, now that I know the kind of questions you ask.

C: In the meantime would you fill in this questionnaire?

RP: Is there anything else you would like me to do before next time?

C: Yes, you can read this book on premature ejaculation and perhaps next time we can discuss what you think of it.

Explaining sensate focus to a man with premature ejaculation

Construct

The candidate must be able to explain the purpose of sensate focus in plain language appropriate to the client's educational level and cultural context.

Instructions to candidate

You have been referred a patient with premature ejaculation. His girlfriend wants to try sensate focus as a treatment but has had difficulty explaining what it is about to her boyfriend.

Please explain the procedure involved to the client in simple terms.

Key points to be covered

- The candidate must check that the patient does have premature ejaculation rather than excessive expectation or erectile dysfunction. Premature ejaculation and erectile dysfunction are distinguished by the loss of an erection after ejaculation, as opposed to the loss of an erection without ejaculation.
- Check briefly that the patient's physical health is good.
- Explore what he already knows about sensate focus and his expectations of treatment.
- Use simple language and try to suggest comparisons with other activities to illustrate your point.
- Make the language you use appropriate to the patient's educational level.
- Attempt to tailor the discussion to the client's cultural background.
- Introduce the idea of a rating scale to monitor progress.

Suggested approach

Opening

C: Hello. My name is Dr —. I understand your GP has referred you to our clinic to help you with premature ejaculation.

RP: Yes. What?

C: Coming too soon when you have sex.

RP: Yeah, much too soon. My girlfriend, Tess, is livid. The doctor mentioned that we had to do some exercises at home.

Follow-on

C: Is it OK if I ask you a few questions?

RP: Right.

C: When you say that you come too soon, how long can you last?

RP: How do you mean?

C: Are you able to penetrate ... to get inside your partner's vagina before coming?

RP: No, I can't. It's all over before I get anywhere.

C: And you want to do something to help get more control, is that right?

RP: I would of thought that was obvious.

C: Fine. One of the treatments that your doctor mentioned is quite effective for what you have got. It is called sensate focus.

RP: That's it – that's what she wants. She read about it on the internet.

C: Do you know anything about it?

RP: No. That is why I am here. Tess said something about that we would both be doing it. What is it doc?

Content

C: Well, it is a course of exercises, like massage, that you do while, at the same time, you are not allowed to have sex.

RP: How can that help? If you don't practise you won't get better, right?

C: At the moment you are practising failure and that is bad for confidence and ability to relax.

RP: I still don't get it. I want to have sex and you tell me not to!

C: Do you like sport?

RP: Yeah. I follow Arsenal. What's your drift?

C: When they train for a match they do drills and sets of exercises right? They don't spend the whole time playing matches.

RP: OK, I've got your message.

C: Well, this is similar. You don't even try to have sex – you just take turns massaging each other. Tess will tell you whether she likes it and show you what she does like. Then you swap round after about 10 minutes.

RP: Which bits do we do?

C: First just back and stomach.

RP: Not very exciting.

C: That is it – it's not meant to be exciting. You just focus on the sensations.

RP: OK.

C: It's important that you go one step at a time. When you have the knack of the first exercise then you can move on to breasts and buttocks and so on. But it is important not to leap ahead before you have mastered the first stage. Later you do the same with your sex parts.

RP: Sorry, 'sex parts'?

C: Your penis and scrotum and Tess's vagina and clitoris.

RP: OK, sex parts – whatever.

C: When you have both got the hang of that stage the next stage involves inserting your penis without thrusting, until we gradually build up to intercourse.

RP: What a palaver.

Closing

C: Perhaps next time we meet Tess could come along as well? In the meantime, I would be grateful if you could fill in this questionnaire with Tess and try reading this book about premature ejaculation.

Sources

Kaplan, H. S. (1989) *How to Overcome Premature Ejaculation.* New York: Brunnel/Mazel.

Spence, S. H. (1991) *Psychosexual Therapy: A Cognitive–Behavioural Approach.* London: Chapman & Hall.

CHAPTER 13

Capacity, consent, communication

Amanda Hukin

Capacity to consent in the context of a physical illness

Construct

The candidate demonstrates the ability to assess the capacity of a patient to consent to breast surgery in an empathetic manner.

Instructions to candidate

You are the psychiatric ward doctor. Mrs Cynthia Granger, a 52-year-old informal patient, has been an in-patient for the past 3 weeks. She was admitted with a severe depressive episode without psychotic features. Her mental state is much improved. However, during the course of her admission, on routine physical examination a breast lump was found. A mammogram indicated a breast carcinoma. She has been seen by the breast surgeons, who have recommended surgery, but she does not wish to have the operation.

Please assess this woman's capacity with regard to her decision to refuse surgery.

Key points to be covered

- Remember that a person is normally assumed to have capacity, that it depends on the subject of the decision and that it can change over time.
- You would normally liaise with the surgeons to determine what stage the cancer is at, what the risks are, what the prognosis would be after the surgery and the risks of the procedure. This of course would not be possible at an OSCE station, but it should be done in routine clinical practice; it ought to be possible at the

station to clarify with the patient what information the surgeons have already given her.

- Assess whether the patient understands the relevant information, is able to retain and believe the information, and is able to make an informed decision.
- She should understand why surgery is being recommended, what is involved in the procedure, the likely risks and benefits, and the likely consequences of declining the treatment.
- If the client lacks capacity, ascertain whether a mental disorder is responsible for this.
- Explore why the patient is refusing to have the operation. There may be many reasons – for example delusions, fear, denial. She may have been given inadequate information; alternatively, she may indeed have made an informed decision and have the capacity to do so.

Suggested approach

Opening
C: Hello Mrs Granger. I'm Dr —.How are you feeling today?
RP: Not too bad; a bit better.
C: Could I talk to you about this operation that's been proposed?
RP: Yes. I don't want it. I don't know if it will do any good.

Follow-on
C: Could I check what you understand to be the problem? What have the doctors told you?
RP: Yes. I believe I have cancer of the breast.

Content
C: What do you understand by cancer?
RP: I believe you may die and it can't be cured. I may need to have an operation to have my breast removed.

Explore what the patient understands by cancer by using appropriate probes.

C: What stage is it in?
RP: I understand it is still in the breast and has not spread to the rest of the body.
C: What would happen if the operation is not carried out?
RP: I don't know. I just don't want an operation.

Assess in detail the patient's understanding, retention of information, belief of the nature and effects of the intervention (in this case surgery) and alternatives, by asking appropriate questions. You could use the following probes: 'What is involved in the operation?', 'What do you see as the benefits of having the operation?', 'What problems do you anticipate?'. It is important, of course, not ask more than one question at a time!

C: Was there any particular reason that you didn't want the operation?
RP: Seems a bit pointless.
C: What do you mean, pointless?
RP: I don't think I will survive anyway.
C: Is it possible the operation will prolong the chances of living a few more years?
RP: I don't know if it will.

Once you have done this check for any underlying mental illness.

Closing

C: We have been discussing your understanding of the diagnosis made by the breast surgeons, the advantages and disadvantages of having the surgery suggested by the surgeons and how it will improve your chances of a more normal life if you have it. Even though you understand the diagnosis and believe you may have cancer, you feel there are far more negatives than positives in having the operation and are not convinced that having the operation may be better in the long term?
RP: Yes.

Source

Bellhouse, J., Holland, A., Clare, I., *et al* (2001) Decision-making capacity in adults: its assessment in clinical practice. *Advances in Psychiatric Treatment*, **7**, 294–301.

Consent for electroconvulsive therapy

Construct

The candidate demonstrates the ability to establish a rapport and attempts to obtain informed consent for ECT from a patient. The candidate should explain why this treatment is being proposed, its nature and the procedure, the possible side-effects and the benefits, in a way that the patient is able to understand.

Instructions to candidate

You are the ward doctor. Mrs Gwyneth Price is a 74-year-old woman who has been an informal in-patient on your ward for the past 2 weeks. This is her first in-patient admission. She has had one previous episode of depression 10 years ago, which was successfully treated with antidepressants. She is now being treated for a severe depressive episode that has not responded to antidepressants. She has been depressed for the past 3–4 months and has had two different antidepressants, but shown little response. Her appetite is poor and she has lost a considerable amount of weight. She has nihilistic delusions.

From the management round it is proposed to treat her with ECT. Please explain the proposed plan and try to obtain consent for this.

Key points to be covered

- Use plain language and check understanding as you proceed
- Assess the patient's baseline knowledge of the treatment and build on this.
- Attempt to obtain informed consent. Valid consent implies the patient understands the nature, purpose and effect of the proposed treatment and the consequences of both having and not having it. The consent should be obtained in an atmosphere free of fear or intimidation and patient should understand that she can withdraw the treatment at any time.
- Do not overemphasise the benefits or understate the risks – it would be helpful to have some facts and figures to ensure that objective information is presented.
- Explain why ECT is being proposed, the procedure (anaesthesia and electric current), the common side-effects (short-term memory loss and headaches) and risks (those of brief general anaesthesia).

- Note that many people have a very negative view of ECT, which has been perpetuated by the media, and may see it a barbaric or punitive form of treatment, hence the importance of providing balanced information in a realistic but non-threatening manner.

Suggested approach

Opening

C: Hello, Mrs Price. How are you today?

RP: About the same.

C: As you are aware, you have been unwell for 3 or 4 months now, and have not been feeling much better. We are wondering whether a new treatment would help. Would you mind if I discuss this in detail with you. Is that alright?

RP: That's fine.

Follow-on

C: The treatment we are considering is called ECT, or electro-convulsive therapy. Have you heard about it?

RP: Yes. Is this the same as shock treatment? You get this when nothing else works. Have I done something wrong?

C: No, you've certainly done nothing wrong. This is just a different sort of treatment that we hope will help you feel better. It is sometimes called shock treatment but there are a lot of mis-understandings about it. It might be helpful if we discussed exactly what it involves, so you can make up your own mind.

Content

C: Well, ECT or electroconvulsive treatment involves you being put to sleep with an anaesthetic, just as if you were getting a minor operation like having your tonsils out. When you are fully asleep, a tiny amount of current is passed across your head. This causes you to have a fit, or seizure. We believe that the seizure changes the chemicals in the brain and leads to an improvement in depression.

RP: Would it hurt? Sounds as if it might, if you are getting an electric shock.

C: It does sound scary but in actual reality you would be fast asleep and not feel any pain – just like the anaesthetic for an operation. Also, the amount of current passed is very small.

RP: Well, I don't like the sound of this 'seizure'.

C: Actually, as well as the anaesthetic, we also give you something to relax your muscles, so the seizure itself is very mild. Your muscles will be so relaxed they will only twitch a bit, for a matter of seconds, less than a minute.

RP: And how many times would I need to have it?

C: Usually we give ECT twice a week. The number of sessions depends on how you respond to the treatment. Some people require more, others less, but six to eight sessions is sort of average, and 12 is as much as we would usually give in one course of treatment.

RP: Do you think it would help my depression?

C: Considering that you have been on medication that hasn't helped yet, it is certainly worth trying. ECT is one of the treatments that often works more quickly than tablets, particularly for your sort of depression, and we would be able to tell if it's working quite soon.

RP: Are there any side-effects? I wouldn't end up like a 'vegetable' would I?

C: Certainly not, but, like most treatments, it does have side-effects, which you are right to ask about. The commonest one is temporary memory problems. You might tend to forget things – especially things that happened on the day of the treatment and the day before. These memory problems seem to be short term and shouldn't persist once the treatment is finished. Headache is another common side-effect, often when people wake up after the treatment, but this can be easily treated as you would any headache, with paracetamol.

RP: The memory problems are worrying

C: I can understand they sound worrying but, as I mentioned before, they tend to get better in a few weeks.

Closing

C: Mrs Price, we have briefly discussed the new treatment, ECT, which we are considering giving you. We talked about the procedure, side-effects and how this treatment can help you. Do you have any questions?

RP: I'm still unsure. Can I think about it?

C: Of course, please do and discuss it with your family and the staff as well. Remember, even if you do decide to have it, you can always change your mind again afterwards. I will give you some leaflets to read and maybe we can have another chat about this in a few days.

RP: That would be better. Thank you very much.

Sources

Lock, T. (1994) Advances in the practice of electroconvulsive therapy. *Advances in Psychiatric Treatment*, 1, 47–56.

Royal College of Psychiatrists' Special Committee on ECT (1994) *Official Video Teaching Pack*. London: Royal College of Psychiatrists.

Explaining the use of a section of the Mental Health Act to a relative

Note that in an OSCE station you are likely to be given instructions that do *not* include the specific number of the section, as mental health legislation varies throughout the territories covered by the College's examination, so look out for terms such as 'for assessment' or 'for treatment'.

Construct

The candidate demonstrates familiarity with and use of the Mental Health Act. The candidate should be able to communicate this to a relative in a sensitive but realistic manner, giving information at an appropriately pitched level.

Instructions to candidate

Mrs Barbara Wilton has requested to speak to you about her son Kelvin, a 20-year-old, single, second-year engineering student who was admitted 2 days ago from student halls following an assessment under the terms of the Mental Health Act. This is his first admission and contact with mental health services. He is acutely psychotic and suicidal. He has marked persecutory delusions and second-person auditory hallucinations, including command hallucinations. There is evidence of self-neglect. He has no insight. He has been detained under section 2 of the Mental Health Act.

You are the ward doctor. His mother wants to know why her son has been detained and what this means. Kelvin has agreed to you talking to his mother.

Please discuss the use of Mental Health Act with his mother.

Key points to be covered

- Remember that this is the patient's first contact with mental health services: his mother is likely to be anxious and worried.
- She may or may not have much knowledge of mental illness or detention, so you should ascertain briefly her knowledge of mental illness and the Mental Health Act.
- Pitch the discussion at her level and check her understanding at every stage.

- Explain the procedures, purpose and nature of the Mental Health Act, including rights of appeal. Even though the patient is on an assessment section, you may need to discuss a possible treatment section.
- Allow time for questions and use simple language – avoid jargon.
- Address the possible implications of the use of the section.
- There is a danger in this scenario of concentrating on the illness and prognosis, and not covering the actual task in the instruction.

Suggested approach

Opening

C: Hello Mrs Wilton, I'm Dr —. I understand that you would like to talk to me about your son Kelvin.

RP: Yes. I'm very worried about him. I only learnt that my son had been admitted yesterday and I drove up last night to see him. The nurse said something about him being sectioned. What is that?

C: Before I go into the details of the section, could I check if you had any concerns about his health before he was admitted to hospital?

Follow-on

Try to establish how much the mother is aware of his illness before explaining the Mental Health Act, but beware of spending too much time on a history, as that is not the task in this scenario.

C: I was wondering whether you've had a chance to see Kelvin yet?

RP: I tried to but he didn't want to see me. He stormed out of the room after only a couple of minutes. It wasn't like Kelvin at all.

C: Oh! That must have been very upsetting for you.

RP: Well, yes.

C: Did you observe any change in his behaviour?

RP: He has seemed a bit preoccupied and did not want to see us. I didn't think too much of it at first, but perhaps if I'd paid more attention maybe this would not have happened.

C: Could you give me an example of a situation when he behaved oddly?

Content

Once you have established her knowledge of the situation, then discuss the Mental Health Act with Mrs Wilton. Check her understanding and give her opportunities to ask questions.

C: It sounds as if you've been quite worried about your son and we became concerned when his GP contacted us. We arranged to see him at his halls and the team felt that Kelvin needed to be in hospital. They were concerned about his health and safety and believed that he might have a mental health problem.

RP: Did he agree to take treatment?

C: I am afraid he did not see the need to take any medicines.

RP: Did you have to bring him to hospital? Could you not have left him at home for another day or two? He might have changed his mind.

C: Unfortunately, Kelvin did not want to come into hospital, but the team decided that it was in his best interests, and that it would be too risky to wait much longer. At the time we did not believe that he was well enough to make this decision for himself.

RP: How would it be possible for one doctor to decide to put someone in hospital against their will?

C: Actually, three people are involved in making that sort of a decision – two independent doctors, one of whom should preferably know him already, and a social worker who has special training in the Mental Health Act. The section would only be completed if all three agreed to this decision.

RP: What section is he on?

Explain about the section for assessment (you may use the section numbers you are familiar with), possible treatment section, appeal procedure, the rights of patients and relatives and so on.

Closing

RP: So he's going to be in hospital for a month?

C: Well, it all depends on how Kelvin is. If he gets better quickly, he may not be in hospital for the whole 28 days, or he may require a longer time in hospital, either as a voluntary patient or still under section, but at this stage it is too early to say. ...

C: Well, I hope that I've managed to answer most of your questions. There is a lot to take in – you might find it helpful to read these leaflets on what we've been discussing today. If you would like to meet up again, please don't hesitate to ask.

Sources

Bethlem and Maudsley NHS Trust (1999) *The Maze: Mental Health Act 1983 Guidelines* (revised 1999). London: Bethlem and Maudsley NHS Trust.

Jones, R. M. (2003) *Mental Health Act Manual* (8th edn). London: Sweet & Maxwell.

Variations

A similar scenario could involve explaining the Mental Health Act to a patient or explaining other detention orders to a patient or relative.

Communication with a colleague

This scenario is an example of a paired station – you assess the patient in one station and communicate your findings in the next. For the purposes of this scenario, assume that you have just completed the first station, which involved gleaning from a medical senior house officer the history of an elderly man on the medical ward who became agitated and struck a nurse with his walking stick, and who, you believe from the available information, is suffering from delirium related to a chest infection.

Construct

The candidate demonstrates the ability to communicate with a senior colleague salient findings from a previous assessment. The candidate highlights the key issues in diagnosis and risk in order to formulate an appropriate immediate management plan.

Instructions to candidate

You are the senior house officer on call for psychiatry in a district general hospital. You have just assessed Mr Albert Wilson, a 72-year-old man who was admitted 5 days ago with a chest infection and acute exacerbation of his chronic obstructive airways disease. Over the past 24 hours he has become increasingly agitated and aggressive. He has struck one of the nurses with his walking stick and is demanding to leave.

Please assess the situation and communicate your findings to your consultant on call by telephone, with a view to making a decision regarding immediate management.

Key points to be covered

From the first station:

- Ideally, clarify the history from the notes and nursers' behaviour reports.
- Interview the patient.
- Explore the risk issues in detail and draw up a short-term management plan. This will depend on the diagnosis, setting, required investigations and level of risk.

In the second station:

- Communicate a summary of the factual findings on the patient's history and mental state.
- Interpret the findings in the context of a diagnostic formulation.
- Discuss all the factors relevant to the risk assessment.
- Highlight the areas that need more detailed information and the investigations needed to confirm the diagnosis.
- State your view on the management, based on the assessment.

Suggested approach (for second station)

Opening

C: Hello, this is Dr —, the on-call psychiatry senior house officer. I wanted to discuss my assessment of Mr Wilson.

E: Yes. What have we got here?

C: Mr Wilson is a 72-year-old male living alone, who has a history of chronic obstructive airways disease and who was admitted for a relapse of his chest infection.

Follow-on

C: He currently appears confused and is agitated on the ward.

E: What are the nurses concerned about?

C: Well, he hit one of the nurses with his walking stick when they tried to stop him leaving the ward.

E: What are the other risk factors?

C: He has a history of alcohol misuse but has no previous history of violence.

Content

E: What is your differential diagnosis?

C: The most likely one is an acute confusional state, the cause of which is unclear.

E: What can we do to clarify the diagnosis?

C: We need to perform [some specified] investigations, get a history from the nearest relative, get the general practitioner's notes and old hospital records. ...

E: With the available information, what would you like to do?

C: He clearly needs further assessment as an in-patient; he may be depressed and could also be in withdrawal.

E: Could we let him go home?

C. In view of his confused state and the risk he poses to others, I would consider using the Mental Health Act in this patient.

E: Which section would you consider?

C: Given the fact that he came informally, has symptoms of mental illness and wants to leave the hospital, we could consider using section 5(2).

Closing

E: Could the medics not use common law to treat him?

C: As there is a history suggestive of depression and current evidence of confusion with an element of risk to others, we could use the Mental Health Act.

E: That is fine. We will go for section 5(2) now, but could you inform the approved social worker that we may need to assess him for a section 2 tomorrow please?

C: Will do. Thanks for your help.

Variations

You may be asked to communicate with a different type of colleague, for example a nurse on a medical ward, in which case you would have to pitch the information appropriately.

CHAPTER 14

Neurological examination

Anish Bahra

In a clinical setting, the scenarios presented in this chapter would take more than 7 minutes to complete. At the OSCE station you would be asked to complete only part of the task, for example to examine the eyes (cranial nerves II, IV, VI) or lower limbs or upper limbs.

Note that in the OSCEs undertaken by physicians and neurologists, candidates are asked to present the relevant findings to the examiner. However, for the MRCPsych examination you are likely to be asked to explain your actions to the examiner as you go along, or the examiner will only observe you doing this. The instructions should clarify this. In the MRCPsych examination you are more likely to get a role-player with no pathology. If you have an anatomical model, you should speak to it as though it were a person.

Examination of the cranial nerves

Construct

The candidate demonstrates a professional and courteous approach to the patient and accurately examines cranial nerves I–XII with a familiarity that would be expected in someone used to performing this examination as part of everyday clinical practice. The candidate should explain all actions for the examiner's benefit.

Instructions to candidate

This 44-year-old woman has been referred by her GP with a 3-week history of drooping right eyelid, diplopia and slurred speech, which tend to worsen later in the day.

Please examine the cranial nerves and give feedback to the patient about your findings. (Fundoscopy is not required.)

Key points to be covered

- Introduce yourself, explain the purpose of the examination and gain the patient's consent to be examined.
- First look for any obvious signs on inspection.
- Examine the cranial nerves sequentially from I to XII.

Suggested approach

Opening

C: Hello. My name is Dr —. I have had a letter from your GP about your recent problems with your eyes and speech. Would you mind if I examined you?'

Inspection

On inspection the patient appears comfortable at rest. There is a right-sided partial ptosis. There is a mild right esotropia. The nasolabial fold appears smoother on the right than on the left.

Examination

Examine the cranial nerves systematically (see Appendix 1 to this chapter). Your instructions may be more specific – for example, examine this patient's lower cranial nerves (V–XII) or eye movements (nerves III–VI).

Response

On examination of the cranial nerves, this patient has a right-sided ptosis. This is fatiguable. There is impaired right abduction of eye movement. There is bilateral upper and lower facial weakness, more marked on the right. The patient is dysarthric. There is a nasal intonation to the speech. On asking the patient to count to 100 the speech became more dysarthric, suggesting fatiguability. There is impaired elevation of the soft palate. There is weakness of neck flexion and bilateral lateral rotation of the neck. In view of the fatiguability the findings would be consistent with a diagnosis of myasthenia gravis.

Fundoscopy

In the MRCPsych examination you will normally have an anatomical model on which to perform fundoscopy, but you should aim to communicate with this as you would with a real person.

Construct

The candidate demonstrates the ability to use a fundoscope in a clinical setting, and sensitively communicates to the patient the procedure and rationale for this form of examination. The candidate will also be expected to describe accurately the factual pathological findings on examination, including the diagnosis, to the examiner.

Instructions to candidate

You have been referred a 28-year-old woman who presents with headache and fleeting visual disturbance, the latter particularly when bending forwards. The patient is comfortable at rest. She is notably overweight.

Please examine the fundi. Explain what you are doing to the patient. Once you have finished the procedure, please explain your findings to the examiner.

Key points to be covered

- Introduce yourself, explain the purpose of the examination and gain the patient's consent to be examined.
- Explain to the patient that you are going to examine the back of each eye with an ophthalmoscope.
- Ensure that the light is switched on and at the start of the examination that the settings are at zero. These can be altered during the examination as required to obtain a clear view of the target.
- Address the examination of the lens, optic disc, vessels, retina and macula.
- Examine each eye in turn.
- Present the findings at the end and give your diagnosis.

Suggested approach

Opening

C: My name is Dr —. Your GP has written regarding your recent headaches and visual problems. Would you mind if I had a look at the back of the eyes?

Examination

See Appendix 1 to this chapter.

Response

The discs are swollen bilaterally as indicated by indistinct disc margins. The vessels are engorged with flame-shaped haemorrhages adjacent to the disc. Venous pulsation is absent. There are a few hard exudates and retinal infarcts. The findings would be consistent with papilloedema.

E: What other findings on the cranial nerve examination would support this diagnosis?.

C: The patient would have preserved visual acuity, restricted peripheral visual fields, an enlarged blind spot and normal pupillary responses.

E: What causes of papilloedema would you want to address?

C: I would first like to perform imaging to rule out a space-occupying lesion that is causing obstructive hydrocephalus or a venous sinus thrombosis. If the imaging is normal, with no evidence of raised pressure, I would measure the pressure of the cerebrospinal fluid and ensure that the constituents are normal. In this situation raised pressure would support a diagnosis of idiopathic intracranial hypertension.

Other fundoscopic characteristics

- *Diabetic retinopathy* – microaneurysms, discrete intraretinal 'dot and blot' haemorrhages and hard exudates. There may be a fine mesh of new vessel formation around the optic disc and surface of the retina adjacent to the retinal vessels.
- *Hypertensive retinopathy* – 'silver wiring' appearance of the arterioles with constriction of the veins at the arteriovenous crossings (arteriovenous nipping). In more progressive disease there may be retinal infarcts ('soft exudates'), retinal haemorrhages radiating from the optic disc and hard exudates forming a partial or complete star around the macula. There may be accompanying papilloedema in patients with malignant hypertension.
- *Optic atrophy* – there is pallor of the optic disc and attenuation of the retinal vessels. If the findings are subtle, a pathological disc can be confirmed by accompanying change in visual acuity, colour vision, visual field (central scotoma) and abnormally slow pupil reactions.
- *Retinitis pigmentosa* – pigmentary retinal degeneration resulting in clumps of pigment in a 'bone corpuscle' pattern. The retinal vessels are attenuated and the optic disc is pale. There is progressive loss of peripheral vision, resulting in 'tunnel vision' and ultimately blindness.

Examination of the extrapyramidal system

Construct

The candidate demonstrates the ability to conduct a competent examination of the extrapyramidal system in a professional and courteous manner.

Instructions to candidate

You are a senior house officer on the ward and have been asked to assess an in-patient who has recently been started on antipsychotic medication. He has been moving more slowly than usual and there has been a change in nature of his speech, which has made his conversation more difficult to understand. The nursing staff felt he may be experiencing extrapyramidal side-effects and are wondering whether his medication regimen needs to be reassessed.

Please examine the patient specifically for any extrapyramidal syndrome, while giving feedback to the patient as you go along.

Key points to be covered

- Introduce yourself, explain the purpose of the examination and gain the patient's consent to be examined.
- Explain that you would like to examine him walking first, and then to examine his arms, legs and speech.
- Assess the patient's gait.
- Look for tremor.
- Demonstrate the additional main features of a Parkinsonian syndrome – rigidity and bradykinesia, dysarthria and impaired writing.
- State to the examiner that you would look for any additional signs to address the range of different Parkinsonian symptoms, such as progressive supranuclear gaze palsy or a multi-system atrophy. Thus examine the eye movements, and look for cerebellar and upper-motor-neuron signs. Look for evidence of autonomic dysfunction, such as a postural blood pressure drop.

Suggested approach

Opening

C: My name is Dr —. I have been asked by the nursing staff to have a look at you. They have been concerned that it has been more difficult for you recently getting in and out of bed and getting dressed. It seems to be taking a longer time for you to do most things. Would you mind if I have a look first at your walking, then your arms and legs? I may also need to perform a few additional tests and check your blood pressure.

Inspection

At rest the patient has an expressionless face. There is no visible rest tremor.

Examination

The approach suggested is set out in Appendix 2 to this chapter.

Response

C: The patient walks with a stooped posture. There is reduced arm swing bilaterally. The gait is narrow-based and short-strided, and has a shuffling appearance. He has some difficulty in turning, and in stopping once he has gained momentum. He is able to walk heel-to-toe, which suggests there is no ataxic component to the gait. The patient has an expressionless appearance. Speech is low in volume and monotonous. There is no tremor. The patient has rigidity and bradykinesia of both the upper and lower limbs. Handwriting is small and untidy. These signs are consistent with a Parkinsonian syndrome. I would further examine for additional features, for example: the eye movements, to look for a supra-nuclear gaze palsy; upper-motor-neuron and cerebellar signs; the lying and standing blood pressure, with regard to a diagnosis of a multi-system atrophy. In the absence of these signs and in view of the recent initiation of antipsychotic medication, an iatrogenic Parkinsonian syndrome would be at the top of my list of differential diagnoses.

Examination of the motor and sensory system

In the MRCPsych examination you are likely to get a normal patient with no neurological findings. Alternatively, the patient may have a history suggestive of conversion disorder, and will display correspondingly variable and physiologically incongruent findings.

Construct

The candidate demonstrates a professional and courteous approach to the patient and accurately examines the motor system and sensory system with a familiarity that would be expected of someone used to performing this examination as part of everyday clinical practice. The candidate should explain all actions to the patient during the examination, for the examiner's benefit.

Instructions to candidate

Mr Smith was referred by his GP as he has developed difficulty walking. You have taken the history and have reached the stage where you need to examine the patient.

Please conduct a neurological examination of the motor and sensory system, using the equipment available as necessary, explaining to the patient your actions as you go along.

Key points to be covered

- Introduce yourself, explain the purpose of the examination and gain the patient's consent to be examined.
- Explain that you would first like to watch the patient walk and then have a look at the arms and legs.
- First make sure you inspect the patient. This should be followed by examination of the gait, the motor system, and the sensory system at the end.

Suggested approach

C: My name is Dr —. Your GP has sent a letter to us regarding your difficulty in walking. I would like to see you walk and then examine your arms and legs, to see whether we can find out what the problem may be.

Inspection

The patient is comfortable at rest and is seated with both legs held in extension and adduction. Inspection and examination of gait give a number of clues. Therefore take time simply to observe the patient and examine the character of the gait.

- Note whether the patient uses a walking aid.
- Are there any additional aids (e.g. ankle splints)?
- Look at the patient's posture – for example, if the patient has hemiparesis, characteristically the upper limb will be held flexed and pronated, and the lower limb extended and adducted.
- Is there any limb deformity? Look for pes cavus (long-standing, usually hereditary, neuropathy) and asymmetrical limb length (as in childhood polio or any other cause of asymmetrical childhood limb paresis).
- Is there any wasting and if so which muscle groups are mainly affected? Is it the distal or proximal muscles, or a localised group of muscles? Is the wasting unilateral or bilateral, symmetrical or asymmetrical?
- Are there fasciculations (present in disorders of the anterior horn or nerves)? These should be observed with the patient adequately exposed and at rest. Movement-related fasciculations are not necessarily pathological. Calf fasciculations are not uncommon, particularly with age.

Examination

The examination of the motor and sensory system is set out in Appendix 3.

Response

The patient is able to walk independently, albeit with difficulty. The gait is stiff, with the lower limbs adducted, giving a scissoring appearance to the gait. Examination of the upper limbs is normal. In the lower limbs there is increased tone, with ankle clonus bilaterally. There is mild weakness bilaterally affecting the flexor muscles more than the extensor muscles. Reflexes are brisk and plantar responses extensor. There is subtle heel–shin ataxia, however; the patient is weak proximally, which may account for this. There is a sensory level for all modalities at T10. Thus this is suggestive of a lesion of the spinal cord at least at T10 or a few levels above this.

Source

Guarantors of Brain (2000) *Aid to Examination of the Peripheral Nervous System*. London: W. B. Saunders.

Appendix 1. Systematic examination of the cranial nerves

I. Olfactory nerve

Unilateral loss of smell is usually asymptomatic. Bilateral loss of smell is not uncommon and most often secondary to pathology of the upper respiratory tract (e.g. chronic rhinitis), heavy smoking or previous head injury. Frontal lobe tumours affecting the olfactory groove (e.g. a meningioma) may also cause a loss of smell. Ask the patient if she has experienced any recent change in her sense of smell. Test each side separately using a series of objects with a characteristic smell (e.g. peppermint, coffee – these would be provided at the station). Ask the patient to name each smell.

II. Optic nerve

Visual acuity

- The patient is made to stand 6 m from a standard Snellen chart. Any refractive error is corrected for, either with glasses or a pinhole.
- Each eye is tested in turn. Visual acuity is expressed as the ratio of the distance between the patient and the number of the smallest visible line on the chart (6/4). If the patient cannot read the characters of the top line (6/60), assess the ability to count fingers, appreciate hand movements or perceive light (with a pen torch). If the latter cannot be discerned, the patient is blind in that eye.
- Near vision is an assessed using a reading chart. Near and distance vision do not always correlate.

Visual fields

- Sit about 1 m from the patient with eyes at the same level. Ask the patient to look at your nose. Test the four quadrants of each visual field by confrontation. Move your finger (peripherally to centrally) in each quadrant with your hand held halfway between you and the patient. Test each eye and quadrant separately; ask the patient to cover the eye not being tested and cover your own corresponding eye.
- Check for visual inattention – test the upper and then lower quadrants, right and left, simultaneously. If there is visual inattention, the patient will perceive movement on each side when tested independently but will not perceive (or attend to) movement on the affected side (lesion in the contralateral, usually non-dominant, parietal cortex).

- Check the blind spot using a 10 mm red hatpin. Cover each eye in turn and test the uncovered eye by comparing this with your own. Bring the pin along the horizontal meridian in a temporal to nasal direction. Explain that the pin will briefly disappear and ensure the patient focuses straight ahead. Once the pin disappears map this horizontally and vertically with your own blind spot.
- The central field can be tested by continuing along the horizontal meridian nasally. If the pin disappears at the point of central fixation, the patient has a central scotoma. This may extend temporally from fixation into the region of the blind spot (centro-caecal).
- Test colour vision with Ishihara plates, for each eye in turn. Colour vision is normal if 13/15 plates at least are read correctly. The test primarily detects congenital abnormalities of colour vision but can pick up optic nerve dysfunction.

Fundoscopy

In dimmed lighting, ask the patient to fixate on a distant target. Examine the right fundus with your right eye and the left with your left eye. Keep both your eyes open. If you wear glasses, these can be kept on or (if easier) taken off; the ophthalmoscope settings can then be changed to allow for not only the patient's but your own refractive error. Stand 1 m from the patient and ensure that the ophthalmoscope settings are at zero. Look through the aperture at the pupils. A red reflex should be seen (this will be absent in a patient with a cataract, for example).

Bring your eye closer to the patient's eye and alter the ophthalmoscope lens setting so that the retinal vessels are in focus. Trace them back to the optic disc. Assess whether the disc margins are distinct. Assess the disc colour. Temporal margins are usually paler than the nasal margins. Physiological cupping varies but does not extend to the disc margins. Look at the arteriole and veins, the arteries are narrower and brighter. Look for venous pulsation, best seen at the disc margins where the veins cross the arteries. Venous pulsation indicates normal intracranial pressure but it is not present in all individuals with a normal pressure. Look for arteriovenous nipping and vessel tortuosity. Look for any haemorrhages, hard exudates, retinal infarcts and pigmentation (e.g. retinitis pigmentosa). Ask the patient to look at the ophthalmoscope light; this should bring the macula into view.

III,IV,VI. Oculomotor, trochlear and abducens nerves, respectively

Pupils: light response

- Check for pupil asymmetry. Test for the direct (ipsilateral) and consensual (contralateral) pupil reflexes using a pen torch. Twenty per cent of individuals have aniscoria (pupil asymmetry) but the pupil responses are normal. In normal pupils when you shine a light in one eye the ipsilateral and contralateral pupil will constrict.

- In an efferent pupillary defect (parasympathetic and thus sphincter pupillae paralysis – fibres carried from the midbrain in the third nerve) the pupil on the affected side will be dilated and unreactive to light. There may also be ophthalmoplegia of the muscles innervated by the third nerve.
- To test for the presence of an afferent pupillary defect, swing the light from one eye to the other. With, for example, a left afferent pupillary defect, on shining the light in the right eye (unaffected) both pupils will constrict promptly; on swinging the light across to the left eye the left pupil will take time to constrict, as there is impairment of optic nerve function on that side. It will initially dilate once the light source on the right is taken away and therefore freed from the consensual response.

Pupils: accommodation

Hold your finger about 50 cm away from the patient and then bring it towards the patient's nose, ensuring that the patient is fixating throughout on the finger. There should be bilateral pupillary constriction and convergence (adduction) of each eye.

Eyelids

Check for a ptosis. Most are incomplete (congenital, mechanical, neurogenic, myopathic). A complete ptosis is usually seen when there is a lesion of the third nerve. If suggested by the history, fatiguability can be tested by asking the patient to look upwards at a target (such as your finger) for 2 minutes. Gradually the ptosis will become more pronounced.

Strabismus/squint

An esotropia is essentially a convergent squint, and an exotropia a divergent squint. A squint can be either paretic or non-paretic (concomitant). The former is dealt with overleaf under ophthalmoplegia in the section on pursuit eye movements. A non-paretic squint is usually congenital (amblyopia or 'lazy eye'). Features of a non-paretic squint are:

- full range of eye movement
- visual acuity on that side is impaired and cannot be corrected
- the cover test is abnormal (for this test, ask the patient to fixate on an object, e.g. light of a pen torch, and while the patient does so, cover the normal eye – the 'lazy eye' will then move and take up fixation).

Binocular vision develops at 6 months and normal visual development is complete at around 6 years of age. If the patient has a non-paralytic squint, vision is not binocular but the image from the 'lazy eye' is suppressed. Thus the patient does not complain of diplopia. This eye will not develop normal vision unless forced to take up fixation before visual development is complete (i.e. 6 years), thus the basis of patching the normal eye to force the 'lazy eye' to take up fixation from its 'lazy' position and to develop normally. A new-onset squint following development of vision will present as diplopia.

Eye movements

Check vertical and horizontal pursuit and saccadic eye movements.

Pursuit eye movements

- Steady the patient's head with one hand and ask him or her to fixate on the index finger of the other hand. Observe the eye movements throughout the range of binocular vision horizontally and vertically. Look for the smoothness of the eye movements.
- *Nystagmus.* If the eye movements are jerky, this is suggestive of a cerebellar lesion. Nystagmus may be present. This must be differentiated from nystagmoid jerks seen at the end of the range of eye movement, just beyond binocular gaze. Nystagmus may be seen in individuals with long-standing impaired vision (pendular), lesions of the cerebellum (jerky and fast phase towards the side of the lesion), brain-stem (jerky, horizontal, vertical or rotary) and peripheral vestibulum (fast phase to the opposite side to the lesion and rotary, which is fatiguable in benign positional vertigo).
- *Ophthalmoplegia.* Look for any overt ophthalmoplegia. This may or may not conform to muscles innervated by a single nerve (e.g. a muscle or neuromuscular junction disorder, or mechanical restriction). Subtle ophthalmoplegia may manifest by diplopia only (i.e. symptoms but no overt signs of ophthalmoplegia). In this situation identify the maximal separation of images; the false image is displaced furthest in the direction of the affected muscle. If the paretic side is covered in the direction of gaze of the affected muscle, the peripheral image will disappear.

Saccadic eye movements

- With the patient's head fixed ahead, ask the patient to look to the left (or to fixate with eyes a target to the left, such as your finger) and then to the right (to a target such as your thumb). Keep alternating right and left movements on command. Note the velocity and range of movement.
- To differentiate a supranuclear (apraxic) from a nuclear (truly paralysed eye movements) gaze palsy, perform the oculocephalic

reflex. Ask the patient to fixate on your eyes and rotate the patient's head horizontally and then vertically. In supranuclear lesions the reflex is intact, allowing the patient's eyes to remain fixated on yours.

V. Trigeminal nerve

Sensory

- Test light touch and pinprick over the forehead, cheek and chin corresponding to the ophthalmic, maxillary and mandibular branches of the trigeminal nerve. Compare both sides of the face.
- Test the corneal reflex by lightly touching the cornea with a wisp of cotton wool; approach the cornea from the side rather than pre-empting a response by direct forward stimulation. An afferent defect (nerve V lesion) results in a reduced or absent response of the direct and consensual reflex. An efferent defect (nerve VII lesion) results in an impaired or absent response on the side of the facial weakness.

Motor

- Nerve V supplies the muscles of mastication – the temporalis, masseter and pterygoid muscles.
- Inspect for wasting of the temporalis muscle, which results in hollowing of the temple above the zygoma.
- Ask the patient to clench the teeth, and then look at and palpate the bulk of the masseter muscles.
- Ask the patient to open the mouth. Look for any jaw asymmetry. In unilateral ptyerygoid weakness the jaw deviates towards the weak side. Test the power of the ptyerygoids by asking the patient to resist attempts to close the open mouth.
- The jaw jerk is a brain-stem stretch reflex. With the mouth slightly open, place your finger on the apex of the chin and tap with a tendon hammer. The normal response is pterygoid contraction of the jaw (upwards). An absent response is not significant. A brisk response is indicative of an upper motor neuron lesion.

VII. Facial nerve

Sensory

The main sensory component of nerve VII (chorda tympani branch) that can be tested is taste of the anterior two-thirds of the tongue. Test sweet (sugar) and sour (vinegar) alternately, and get the patient to rinse the mouth in between.

Motor

The facial nerve is primarily a motor nerve and supplies the muscles of facial expression. There is bilateral supranuclear innervation to the upper part of the face and unilateral innervation to the lower part of the face. Thus an upper motor neuron lesion will cause weakness of the lower part of the face with sparing of the upper part (furrowing of the brow is preserved, for example). A lower motor neuron lesion will cause weakness of both the upper and lower facial muscles.

- Ask the patient to screw the eyes up tightly and try to overcome this. With good effort, Bell's phenomenon will be present – on attempted eye closure there is reflex upward eye deviation.
- Ask the patient to furrow the brow.
- Ask the patient to smile, and note any facial asymmetry.
- Ask the patient to purse the lips tight and resist your attempt to open them.

Bilateral facial weakness can be easily missed on inspection and will become more apparent on formal testing, as above.

VIII. Vestibulocochlear nerve

Hearing

- Mask one ear by either occluding the external auditory meatus with your index finger or rubbing the finger adjacent to the meatus to produce a distracting sound. About half a metre from the opposite ear (i.e. that to be tested), whisper a number and ask the patient to repeat this. Masking the opposite side will ensure that if the patient is deaf on the side tested he or she will not hear from the unaffected opposite side. If hearing is abnormal, go on to perform the Rinnie and Weber tests.
- With Rinnie's test, the base of a vibrating 512 Hz tuning fork is first held against the mastoid process and then, when the tone has disappeared, about 2.5 cm from the external auditory meatus. Normally air conduction (sound transmitted through the outer and middle ear to the cochlea) is better than that through bone (thus bypassing the middle-ear apparatus). In conductive deafness this ability is impaired by disease of the outer or middle ear, thus bone conduction is better. With sensorineural deafness there is impaired sound perception through air and bone. However, sound may be transmitted through bone to the opposite, unaffected ear, giving a false positive result.
- Weber's test is performed by placing the vibrating tuning fork in the middle of the forehead. The sound should be heard centrally (i.e. equally by both ears). In conductive deafness the sound is

heard by the affected ear. In sensorineural deafness the sound lateralises to the normal ear.

IX, X. Glossopharyngeal and vagus nerves, respectively

The glossopharyngeal nerve is mainly sensory to the palate and taste in the posterior third of the tongue.

- Sensation can be tested by gently touching the posterior pharyngeal wall on the right and left with a wooden applicator stick (an orange stick).
- Taste for sweet and sour in the posterior third of the tongue can be tested as for the anterior tongue.

The vagus nerve provides the motor supply to the pharynx, larynx and palate.

- Ask the patient to say 'aah' and observe the movement of the palate. In the presence of unilateral lower motor neuron lesions, the palate moves towards the unaffected side. Supranuclear innervation is bilateral and therefore the patient will be asymptomatic from a unilateral lesion. In the presence of bilateral upper motor neuron lesions, there may be impaired voluntary palatal movement but a brisk response on performing the gag reflex.

The afferent arm of the gag reflex is subserved by nerve IX and the efferent arm by nerve X.

- Observe the symmetrical rise of the soft palate and movement of the pharyngeal muscles on testing pharyngeal sensation.
- A good test of nerves IX and X is the coordinated act of swallowing. Ask the patient to drink a glass of water. Observe whether the patient aspirates (coughs and splutters).

Weakness of the facial (nerve VII), pharyngeal and laryngeal (nerves IX and X) muscles or tongue muscles (XII) can cause dysarthria.

XI. Accessory nerve

The spinal part of nerve XI is purely motor and arises from the upper five segments of the cervical spinal cord. It supplies the trapezius and sternocleidomastoid muscles.

- Look for wasting of the muscles.
- For the sternocleidomastoid muscle, test the strength of neck flexion (muscles on both sides contract) and right and left lateral rotation of the head (the muscle on the opposite side to rotation contracts).
- For the trapezius muscle, ask the patient to shrug the shoulders, and observe the elevation and strength of the trapezius muscles.

XII. Hypoglossal nerve

This is a purely motor nerve to the muscles of the tongue.

- Look for any wasting and fasiculation of the tongue muscles. The latter is best assessed by observing the tongue at rest on the floor of the open mouth.
- Look at tongue protrusion. With weakness the tongue will deviate towards the affected side. With a spastic tongue (bilateral upper motor neuron lesions which produce a pseudobulbar palsy) the tongue protrusion will be restricted (and jaw jerk brisk).

Appendix 2. Examination of a patient with suspected Parkinsonian syndrome

Gait

Ask the patient to walk, say, 5–10 metres and then to turn round. Assess the following:

- posture (is it stooped?)
- arm swing (is this reduced and if so is this symmetrical or asymmetrical?)
- length of stride (this is reduced in Parkinsonian syndromes)
- stance: is it narrow or wide-based? (patients who are ataxic have a wide-based gait)
- ability to turn.

Then ask the patient to walk heel-to-toe to look for any signs of ataxia. Patients often feel they are unable to do so, thus they may need some encouragement and support during the test, which is then usually performed adequately if they are not ataxic.

Romberg's test addresses proprioceptive function. Ask the patient to stand with feet together. A patient who is ataxic may find this difficult and stand on a wider base. Ask the patient to close the eyes. Wait for about 2 minutes. If there is normal proprioception the patient will maintain balance. If proprioception is impaired, the patient is likely to fall. Again, the patient is likely to need encouragement to persist with the task. A negative test is more reliable than a positive test.

Tremor

A tremor can be present at rest, on postural change or on intention. A rest tremor is characteristic of Parkinson's disease. A postural tremor may be physiological (exacerbated in anxiety), iatrogenic (exacerbated by lithium or alcohol), secondary to a systemic process (e.g. thyrotoxicosis) or a benign essential tremor. An intention tremor is due to ataxia, usually cerebellar in origin.

Rest tremor

To test for a rest tremor, observe the upper limbs at rest at the patient's side. A rest tremor may become more apparent after the upper limb has been exercised (ask the patient to flex and extend the limb at the elbow a few times). A pill-rolling tremor is coarse, worse with anxiety and settles during sleep. It may improve with posture and intention. The lower limb, tongue, lips and chin may be affected.

Postural tremor

Ask the patient to stretch out the arms and hold the fingers apart. A postural tremor may become apparent. The postural characteristic may be brought out by asking the patient then to bring both index fingers towards the nose, but without the fingers touching each other or the nose. In patients with essential tremor the trunk and head may also be affected.

Intention tremor

To elicit an ataxic tremor, ask the patient in turn to touch the nose with the index finger and then to touch your finger, which should be held at arm's length from the patient. Do this a few times; an ataxic tremor will become more apparent, if present. The patient may have a head tremor (titubation) and ataxia of the lower limbs and gait.

Tone

The patient must be relaxed. Examine the tone in the upper limbs at the elbows (in flexion and extension, pronation and supination) and at the wrists (in flexion and extension). Passively flex and extend the knee at varying speeds, supporting both the thigh and the foot. Look for ankle clonus. This will be absent in a pure Parkinsonian syndrome (i.e. without additional upper-motor-neuron features).

In a Parkinsonian syndrome the patient will have increased tone equally in all directions of movement – the characteristic 'lead-pipe rigidity'. In the upper limb this may be more evident on synkinesis – while testing tone in the limb ask the patient to move the opposite limb up and down. If a tremor is present, the tone will take on a 'cogwheel' rigidity.

Bradykinesia

Slowing and paucity of movements affect the whole body. This is manifest in the muscles of facial expression by mask-like facies. There is general difficulty initiating movement (e.g. getting out of a chair or initiating walking). Bradykinesia can be tested in the upper limbs by asking the patient to touch the thumb and index finger of one hand repeatedly. If the patient is bradykinetic, the movements will be slow, and lose speed and amplitude. Both sides should be tested, for evidence of asymmetry.

Speech

The patient's speech will be characteristically hypophonic, monotonous without inflection, and tends to tail off at the end of a sentence. In advanced disease, the speech is often mumbling and unintelligible.

Handwriting

Ask the patient to write a sentence. The handwriting becomes progressively smaller (micrographia) and spidery.

Additional features

- Power is preserved. There may be apparent weakness due to bradykinesia, but given time power will be found to be full.
- Coordination is normal.
- Reflexes are normal and plantar responses flexor. The plantar response may appear to be up-going – the dystonic 'striatal toe'.
- Sensory examination is normal.
- There may be impairment of cognition, which in Parkinson's disease occurs late.

Parkinsonian syndromes

Parkinson's disease

The syndrome is characterised by asymmetry, a predominantly upper (although there may be a lower) limb tremor at rest. Onset is usually insidious and slowly progressive. There is a good symptomatic response to L-dopa.

Iatrogenic

Drug-induced Parkinsonism is characterised by the above clinical features *but* there is an absence of tremor and there is symmetry of signs.

Multi-system atrophy

- *Striatonigral degeneration*. The patient has a Parkinsonian syndrome without tremor and without asymmetry.
- *Shy–Drager syndrome*. There is additional autonomic dysfunction such as orthostatic hypotension. The patient may complain of

urinary frequency, urgency and incontinence, and impotence.
- *Olivopontocerebellar atrophy.* There are additional cerebellar and upper-motor-neuron signs.

Other Parkinsonian syndromes

- *Progressive supranuclear gaze palsy* – restriction of voluntary, primarily vertical gaze, a pseudobulbar palsy and a tendency to fall backwards.
- *Diffuse Lewy-body dementia* – early dementia with prominent visual hallucinations.
- *Wilson's disease* – Kayser–Fleischer rings (there may be dystonia, chorea and/or myoclonus).

Appendix 3. Examination of the motor and sensory system

Gait

The nature of a patient's gait gives many clues to the underlying problem and what you may expect to find on further examination. There are a number of characteristic types of gait:

- *Cerebellar ataxia.* The patient stands and walks with a wide-based stance (i.e. with feet spaced widely apart). The gait is unsteady, with variable stride. The patient is unable to walk heel-to-toe. This may be the only manifestation of an ataxic gait. Romberg's test is negative.
- *Sensory ataxia.* The abnormal gait arises from impaired proprioception. Again, the patient has a wide-based gait. However, the gait is high-stepping and with a 'stamping' quality. Romberg's test is positive.
- *Hemiparetic.* The patient has the posture characteristic of someone with an upper-motor-neuron lesion – upper limb(s) held flexed and pronated and lower limb(s) extended and adducted, with stronger flexors in the upper limbs and extensors in the lower limbs. The lower limb is held stiffly and swung round in a semicircle to avoid the foot scraping the floor. The outer aspect and toe, however, often does scrape and footwear is worn in the corresponding distribution.
- *Spastic.* The patient has either a bilateral hemiparesis or paraparesis. The legs move stiffly and in adduction such that the patient's legs may cross, thus the characteristic scissoring gait.
- *Parkinsonian.* The character of this gait is detailed in Appendix 2.
- *Apraxic.* Pathology of the frontal lobes gives rise to an apraxic gait. Thus on the couch there may be no obvious abnormality on motor

and sensory testing of the lower limbs but when asked to walk the patient cannot do so. There is difficulty initiating walking and when the patient does so the steps are very short-strided and as though the feet are stuck to the ground.

- *Steppage*. This arises from weak pretibial and peroneal muscles. The patient has a dropped foot with inability to dorsiflex and evert the foot. The limb is therefore lifted in an attempt to clear the foot off the ground. On striking the floor again a slapping sound may be heard.
- *Myopathic*. This is due to a disorder of the muscles. A muscle or neuromusular junction disorder usually affects the proximal limb muscles symmetrically. The gait thus has a waddling appearance.
- *Antalgic*. Pain in the limb (e.g. from knee or hip arthritis) gives rise to an antalgic gait. The patient tends to 'hobble', attempting to weight-bear mainly on the unaffected side and briefly on the affected side.
- *Hysterical*. The gait conforms to none of the above and is variable in character.

Assuming the patient is able to walk unaided:

- ask the patient to walk a distance and observe posture, stance and stride, and try to characterise the gait as above;
- ask the patient to turn round and look for any difficulties in doing this;
- ask the patient to walk heel-to-toe;
- perform Romberg's test (Appendix 2).

The motor system

Examination of the motor system includes examination of tone, power, coordination and reflexes.

Tone

The patient must be relaxed.

- Examine the tone in the upper limbs at the elbows (in flexion and extension, pronation and supination) and at the wrists (in flexion and extension). Mild spasticity may be detected as a 'catch' in the pronators on passive pronation/supination of the forearm and in the wrist flexors on flexion/extension.
- Passively flex and extend the knee at varying speeds, while supporting both the thigh and the foot. With the patient's leg extended put your hands under the knee and quickly lift the leg about 20 cm. If hypotonic, the limb will fall laxly like a 'rag doll'. If the tone is increased, it will be stiff and move as one unit. Look for ankle clonus – sudden sustained dorsiflexion of the foot at the

ankle elicits a stretch reflex. While the stretch is maintained there may be unidirectional rhythmic beats of the foot. Two to three beats of clonus are normal. Persistent clonus occurs in the presence of upper-motor-neuron lesions.

The site of different lesions will govern tone (see Table 14.1).

Power

Power should be tested in each of the main muscle groups and graded against resistance applied by the examiner.

Power should be tested in the muscle groups as shown in Table 14.1. Power in each muscle group is graded according to the Medical Research Council scale (Table 14.2).

The characteristic patterns of muscle weakness, according to the site of the lesion, are shown in Table 14.3.

Coordination

In the presence of normal power, the ability to make accurate and smooth movements will depend on coordination. Weakness may give rise to apparent clumsiness, which can be misinterpreted as in-coordination.

The examination of gait has been described above.

For the upper limbs, perform the following:

- *The finger–nose test.* With your finger held at arm's length from the patient, ask the patient to touch your finger with their index finger and then to touch their nose with the same index finger. Ask the patient to do this alternately and as accurately as possible. In a patient with ataxia (e.g. in a cerebellar lesion), as the finger approaches that of the examiner there is a coarse tremor (intention tremor) with over-shooting (past-pointing) of the target (i.e. the examiner's finger).
- *Dysdiadokokinesis.* This is the inability to perform rapid alternating movements. Ask the patient alternately to pronate and supinate the arm and correspondingly tap the palm and dorsum of the hand on the patient's opposite palm. In patients with ataxia the speed, fluency and regularity of movement will be impaired.

For the lower limbs, perform the following:

- *The heel–shin test.* To test the right lower limb ask the patient to put the right heel on the left knee and then run it smoothly down the shin. This should be repeated with the heel lifted off the leg and placed on the knee again (rather than running the heel back up and then down the shin without lifting it off the shin). The left lower limb should be tested similarly. In patients with ataxia the heel does not run down the shin in a straight line but irregularly.

Table 14.1 Motor examination of the limbs

Muscle group	Innervation
Upper limb	
Shoulder abduction (deltoid)	C5
Shoulder adduction (pectoralis major, latissimus dorsi)	C6–7
Elbow flexion (biceps)	C5–6
Elbow extension (triceps)	C7–8
Wrist extension (wrist extensors)	C6–7
Finger extension (finger extensors)	C7–8
Finger flexion (finger flexors)	C8–T1
Finger abduction (dorsal interossei)	
Thumb abduction (abductor pollicis brevis)	C8–T1
Lower limb	
Hip flexion (iliopsoas)	L1–2
Hip extension (gluteus maximus)	L5–S1
Knee flexion (hamstrings)	L5–S1
Knee extension (quadriceps)	L3–L4
Ankle dorsiflexion (tibialis anterior and long extensors)	L4–L5
Plantar flexion (gastrocnemius)	S1–S2

Table 14.2 Medical Research Council scale for grading muscle power

Degree of power	Rating
No movement	0
Flicker of movement	1
Movement but not against gravity	2
Movement against gravity but not resistance	3
Movement against resistance but which can be overcome by the examiner	4
Movement against resistance which cannot be overcome by the examiner	5

Reflexes

- Tendon reflexes are elicited by tapping briskly on, and thus stretching, the tendon with a tendon hammer. The tendon can be tapped either directly or onto a finger placed over the tendon. The reflex may be normal, reduced/elicited with reinforcement, absent or brisk. If a reflex cannot be elicited, it should be tested again with reinforcement. In the upper limbs, as the reflex is being tested the patient is asked simultaneously to clench the teeth and then relax before testing for a reinforced reflex again. In the lower limbs, as the reflex is tested, the patient can be asked to clench the fists.
- The plantar response is elicited by scraping the sole of the foot with an orange stick from just above the heel and laterally,

Table 14.3 Motor examination

Site of lesion responses	Tone	Power	Reflexes	Plantar
Upper motor neuron	Increased	Stronger upper-limb flexors and lower-limb extensors – 'pyramidal pattern weakness'	Brisk	Extensor
Lower motor neuron	Reduced	Individual groups of muscles: Root – weakness only if multiple adjacent roots involved Plexus – weakness of muscles supplied by the affected roots forming the plexus Peripheral nerve – weakness of muscles supplied by a single nerve Peripheral neuropathy – usually length-dependent, therefore with distal muscle weakness	Elicited with reinforcement or absent	Flexor
Neuromuscular junction	Normal	Bilateral, symmetrical, mainly proximal limb girdle – characteristically fatiguable	Normal	Flexor
Muscle	Normal/reduced if severe disease with marked muscle wasting	Bilateral proximal limb girdle	Decreased in proportion to muscle wasting	Flexor
Cerebellar	Normal/reduced	Normal	Pendular	Flexor
Parkinsonian	Increased equally throughout the range of limb movement. No clonus	Normal	Normal	Flexor

upwards, curving round at the top of the foot towards the big toe. A normal response is plantar flexion of the big toe, with fanning out of the other toes. An abnormal response seen in the presence of upper-motor-neuron lesions is dorsiflexion of the big toe. Remember that if toes are weak there may be no movement.

The tendon reflexes are listed in Table 14.4.

The sensory system

Test in a dermatomal pattern, first comparing one side with the other. Ask the patient if each side feels the same. Ask the patient if there is any difference as you progress down the dermatomes proximally to distally. If there is a difference, then test from proximal to distal down the limb to look for a 'glove and stocking' distribution of sensory impairment. If there is focal unilateral sensory impairment, this may be within the distribution of a plexus, roots or a single peripheral nerve, which should then be tested in more detail. Test the modalities carried by the spinothalamic (pinprick and temperature) and dorsal column (light touch, vibration and proprioception) pathways.

For distribution of dermatones and peripheral nerves see Anonymous, 2000. The pattern of sensory loss (if any) will depend on the site of the lesion (if any):

- cerebral hemisphere (cortex, or subcortical–thalamus) – contralateral hemisensory impairment
- brain-stem – ipsilateral face and contralateral limb and trunk impairment
- spinal cord – sensory level depends on the site of the lesion
- roots – dermatomal
- plexus – multiple dermatomes comprising the brachial or the lumbosacral plexus
- peripheral nerve(s).

Pinprick

Use a sensory testing pin, test pain sensation. The patient should be able to differentiate between the sharp and blunt ends of the pin.

Temperature

Cold can be tested using, for example, the flat surface of a non-vibrating tuning fork.

Light touch

Using a wisp of cotton wool. Make sure to avoid tickling the patient, as the spinothalamic fibres carry this modality.

Table 14.4 Tendon reflexes

Reflex	Innervation
Triceps	C7–8
Biceps	C5–6
Supinator	C5–6
Knee	L3–4
Ankle	S1–2
Plantar response	S1

Vibration

Set a 128 Hz vibrating tuning fork against the chin and ask the patient if he or she can feel the fork vibrating. If so, then place the tuning fork on the distal phalanx of the upper limb and then lower limb digit and again ask whether the patient can feel the tuning fork vibrating.

Ideally you should ask the patient to close the eyes and ask when the tuning fork stops vibrating, which should coincide with your stopping the vibration at the tip of the fork. If the vibration cannot be felt, gradually move proximally. Thus, in the lower limb start at the distal phalynx and move to the lateral malleolus, the tibial tuberosity, the external iliac crest and the costal margin. In the upper limb start at the distal phalynx and progress to the wrist, elbow and then shoulder. Stop when vibration is perceived and is comparable to that on the chin.

Proprioception

Start at the distal interphalangeal joint in the upper and then lower limbs. Move the joint of the index finger up or down and show the patient the direction you are moving the digit. Ask the patient to close the eyes. In random sequence move the joint up/down several times, holding the sides of the digit. Ask the patient to indicate in which direction the digit is moving. If there are mistakes, move proximally. In the upper limb, progress to the wrist, then move to the elbow and shoulder on each side in turn, until the patient can correctly identify joint position. In the lower limb, start with the distal interphalyngeal joint of the big toe and if the patient is incorrect move to the ankle, knee and hip.

Sources

Anonymous. (2000) *Aids to the Examination of the Peripheral Nervous System (4th edn)*. Edinburgh: Churchill Livingstone.

CHAPTER 15

Feedback of neurological investigations

Ranga Rao

Feedback of the results of magnetic resonance imaging

Construct

The candidate is expected sympathetically but accurately to communicate the results of a magnetic resonance imaging (MRI) scan to a patient's relative; the explanation should be at an appropriate level and the candidate should check the relative's understanding.

Instructions to candidate

You are a senior house officer working in a general psychiatric ward. A 63-year-old woman who has a diagnosis of schizophrenia with positive symptoms resistant to treatment was noticed to be forgetting names of people and an MRI scan was requested. You have just received the results, which conclude with the following comment: 'vascular changes with lacunar infarcts and mild cortical atrophy in keeping with her years'. Her daughter wants to discuss the scan results with you and the patient has consented to this.

Please convey the results of the MRI scan to the patient's daughter, who is anxious to know the outcome of this investigation.

Key points to be covered

- Remember, any brain scan raises anxieties in both patients and relatives.
- Use plain language and avoid jargon as far as possible.

- Check understanding as you proceed.
- Allow time for questions.
- Convey the factual information without causing alarm.
- Communicate clearly the facts in the report, such as vascular changes and the possibility of strokes in future, and convey the fact that the mild cerebral atrophy could be related to the patient's age.
- Clarify the possible relationship of the findings to the patient's current illness.
- State the long-term prognosis (which is essentially a balance of probabilities).
- Arrange another time to go over this again if the relative finds there is a lot of information to absorb.

Suggested approach

Opening

C: Hello. I'm Dr —. I believe you wanted to talk about your mother's brain scan results?

RP: Yes. I was wondering whether you could tell me what the results of the scan are.

C: As you are probably aware, your mother has been on the ward for a while now and was also having some difficulty remembering things. We wanted to check whether there were any changes in her brain contributing to this.

Follow-on

RP: Yes, she has been on the ward for 3 months now and even though she got better initially, it seems to have remained at the same level for the past few weeks. I heard that she had a brain scan and wanted to check if everything was alright.

C: The scan results arrived this morning and there are one or two things I wanted to discuss with you.

RP: What does it show? Is it something to worry about?

C: First, there are no major problems with the scan.

RP: Oh, that's a relief!

Content

C: However, there are a couple of abnormalities. First, overall her brain appears to have possibly shrunk a little.

RP: What does that mean? Is it like dementia or something?

C: Well, it's commonly an age-related finding, because as we grow older our brains do shrink a bit. Considering that your mother is 63 years old it is possible that these changes may represent a normal ageing process, although it is also something, as you mentioned, that can be seen with things like dementia.

RP: Does that mean that this change will continue to progress?

C: It would be difficult to predict with any degree of confidence when and by how much these changes will deteriorate. It is also possible that they might remain the same for years. ...

C: The scan also indicates that the blood vessels which supply blood to her brain have thickened a bit. As you probably know, if the blood vessels become thicker, the amount of blood that passes through them will actually decrease. Do you understand?

RP: Oh, yes. What would that mean?

C: This means parts of the brain may not have had a fully adequate blood supply, causing some small areas of damage to the brain tissue. These are what have shown up on the scan.

RP: How would that affect her?

C: Well, you may have heard of people having something called a stroke, when a piece of the brain is damaged because of its poor blood supply.

RP: Like, with paralysis and all that?

C: That's what happens when the bigger blood vessels are affected. In your mother's case it appears as if it's the smaller blood vessels, so the individual areas of damage are very small. That's why we haven't seen anything like the paralysis you get with big strokes.

RP: That is reassuring.

C: But it might well account for the difficulty she's been having remembering things recently.

RP: Oh dear. I see ...

Closing

C: So, we have briefly talked about the results of the scan showing that there is an age-related shrinking of the brain and a thickening of the blood vessels. At present this is happening only in the smaller blood vessels and hence tiny parts of her brain have been affected. The question of how quickly these changes may progress will depend on the other factors we have discussed.

RP: Thank you doctor. I will talk to my sister and brother and come back to you if we have any questions – is that alright with you?

C: That would be fine.

Feedback of the results of electroencephalography

Construct

The candidate feeds back the results of electroencephalography in a sensitive manner using appropriate language, and checks the patient's understanding while proceeding.

Instructions to candidate

You are a senior house office seeing Mr Singh, a 30-year-old single male with depression and anger outbursts, for a routine follow-up in the out-patient clinic. On review of his notes there was an electro-encephalogram (EEG) requested by your predecessor to rule out temporal lobe epilepsy (TLE). The report states:

There is evidence of bilateral slow-wave activity, which could be due to the antidepressant medication he is taking; however, there are infrequent bursts of sharp and slow waves, which could not be localised. These findings need to correlated with the clinical picture and referral for further investigation if required.

You have done the routine out-patient review and have come to the point when you need to discuss the results of the EEG with the patient.

Please discuss the EEG report with the patient.

Key points to be covered

- Convey the results without using jargon – use simple language as far as possible.
- Establish the baseline knowledge of the patient.
- Check his understanding as you go along.
- Avoid inducing panic.
- Point out that, unlike a scan that shows you structural brain abnormalities, an EEG is able only to pick up surface electrical activity, which is subject to interpretation.
- Convey the limitations of the EEG and emphasise the need for further investigations to confirm any abnormalities.

Suggested approach

Opening

C: Now, you were sent for a test called an EEG a few weeks ago, weren't you?

RP: Yes, that's right. All those wires on my head. I was wondering if you could tell me what it shows? Is it normal?

Follow-on

C: Well, we have the results here, but, before I discuss them, could I just ask you what you understand to be the reasons for this test?

RP: I used to get angry and 'fly off the handle' sometimes. I thought it was due to my drinking but this continued even after I stopped. Your colleague wanted to check the reasons for this.

C: What do you think the test might show?

RP: Well, I suppose it might tell us why I am getting these anger outbursts and get me some pills to cure this.

Content

C: OK, so in rare cases angry outbursts can be caused by abnormal electrical activity in the brain, and the EEG would test to see if there is any of this in your case.

RP: Do you mean to say that there is some current passing in my brain, which I can feel?

C: The cells in our brain use a minute amount of electricity to communicate with each other. This is quite normal, and is so tiny that we can only pick it up with the electrodes or wires which were put on your head before the recording. An EEG is basically a recording of this activity, which goes on on the surface of your brain.

RP: That is all right then. What does the report show?

C: First, the antidepressant medication you are taking has caused some changes which interfered with the actual recording. This is quite expected.

RP: Would it have been better if I had stopped the medication before the test?

C: That would have been an option, but stopping the medication might have caused other problems, such as your depression getting worse again. So not to worry about that. However, the report also came up with some abnormal recordings.

RP: What does that mean?

C: These are bursts of electrical activity that stand out above the normal activity of the brain. They are sometimes seen in normal people but they are also seen in patients who have fits.

RP: Does that mean I have epilepsy doctor?

C: As I was saying, these abnormalities can also be seen in normal people, but we cannot be sure what is causing them unless we do some more tests. As I mentioned earlier, my colleague arranged this test to see if any abnormal electrical activity might be accounting for your angry episodes. These results suggest that you need more tests for us to be certain what the underlying problems are.

RP: What kind of tests would I need doctor?

C: Well, for a start, we might need to repeat the EEG after stopping the medication you are on for a day or two. If the results are still abnormal, you might need an EEG that it is recorded over a period of 24 hours.

Closing

C: To sum up, we discussed briefly what your EEG report indicates. At present, even though there are no major abnormalities, there are some findings that suggest the need for more tests to see if they might be related to your anger problems. At the end of the day, everything might be quite normal, but we do need to check further. If it's OK, I'll arrange these further tests and see you in a few weeks' time?

RP: Thank you doctor.

Other possible stations:

CPR station

The skill being tested in this station is the ability to perform cardiopulmonary resuscitation. This is usually performed on a manikin. The key aspects to be covered in this station are the need to check responsiveness, call for help, open the airway, check breathing, deliver two effective breaths and check for circulation, before starting CPR as appropriate. You should arrange training with your local resuscitation training officer to help prepare you for the examination, and in any case keep this essential clinical skill up to date.

Use of equipment

A good example of this is electrode placement for ECT. The key aspects to be covered are checking handedness and the electrode placement for unilateral and bilateral ECT. You should get hands-on training from your local consultant responsible for ECT, and be familiar with the materials published by the Royal College of Psychiatrists on this subject.

Index

Compiled by Caroline Sheard